NOVOREADS

VITAMIN E AND LUNG CANCER RISK MODELS

Part of series: Cancer Epidemiology, Research and Theory

Dr. Widad Akreyi

Cover and book design by NovoReads Team

Scientific illustrations by the author (with utilization of keynote)

The author certifies that she does not have any actual or potential conflict of interest, including any financial, consultant, or other relationships with people or institutions, that would inappropriately influence (or bias) her work.

ISBN-13: 978-82-8405-002-7
NovoReads Edition 2018

The author has donated her manuscripts to charities that work to improve the lives of people in need, both locally and internationally.

DEDICATION

To lung cancer patients and their loved ones.

BOOK DESCRIPTION

Lung cancer is considered one of the most common and fatal form of cancer and as such, it requires urgent attention from medical researchers in order to slow its current epidemic proportions. This book analyzes the dose-response relationship of vitamin E intake on the risk of developing lung cancer, with emphasis placed on both dietary and supplemental intakes of vitamin E, as well as the various barriers to identifying the biological processes that drive lung cancer formation. The aim of the book is to improve our understanding of the empirical and mechanism-based vitamin E-lung cancer models, and to aid in developing new strategies for the treatment and prevention of lung cancer. The book sets the stage for a discussion on the dose-response modeling of vitamin E intake and lung cancer risk by briefly describing the concept of dose-response and its quantified strength of association in two selected cohort studies, and by presenting the cellular mechanisms through which vitamin E may exert its anti-cancer activity. Safe and beneficial dietary and supplemental doses of vitamin E are estimated, as are its critical doses. Throughout the book, gaps in knowledge relating to the evaluation of the relationship between vitamin E intake and lung cancer risk, especially those in dose-response analyses, are revealed. Understanding these gaps and their implications can inform the design of new dose-response studies, which may add to our knowledge of vitamin E activity and shed light on issues related to its bioavailability and action in lung cells. The book concludes by summarizing the main conclusions and implications derived from this assessment.

Key words: Lung cancer, vitamin E, empirical dose-response models, mechanism-based dose-response models, COX regression models, public health, cancer epidemiology.

TABLE OF CONTENTS

LIST OF TABLES

LIST OF ABBREVIATION

α-T	Alpha-Tocopherol
Apaf-1	Apoptosis protease-activating factor 1
ASK1	Apoptosis Signal-regulating Kinase 1
BMI	Body Mass Index
Caspase-8	Cysteine Aspartate Specific ProteASE 8
CAD	Caspase-Activated Deoxyribonuclease
CI	Confidence Interval
JNK pathway	c-Jun N-terminal Kinase pathway
DAXX	Death Associated protein 6
DD	Death Domain
DED	Death-Effector Domain
DISC	Death-Inducing Signaling Complex
FADD	Fas-Associated protein with Death Domain
γ-T	Gamma-tocopherol

HRs	Hazard Ratios
hTERT	human TElomerase Reverse Transcriptase
ICAD	Inhibitor Caspase-Activated Deoxyribonuclease
LAP	Latency-Associated Propeptide
LTBP	Latent Transforming growth factor-β Binding Protein
MAP3K5	Mitogen-Activated Protein Kinase Kinase Kinase 5
MAPKs	Mitogen-Activated Protein Kinases
PARP	Poly-ADP-Ribose Polymerase
RR	Relative Risk
STKs	Serine-Threonine Kinases
SMAD3	Mothers Against Decapentaplegic homolog 3
TGF-βs	Transforming Growth Factor-betas
TNF-α	Tumor Necrosis Factor α
XIAP	X-linked Inhibitor of Apoptosis Protein

INTRODUCTION

Abstract

This introduction provides a brief overview of the global and scientific relevance of this topic, how vitamin E has been linked to lung cancer risk, followed by a brief outline of book highlights and key areas, including research questions, covered in this book. It also offers summaries of the two selected studies, one conducted by Slator et al. (2008) and one by Writh et al. (2004) that will be discussed and analyzed in details in the second chapter.

Significance of Topic

Lung cancer is a serious illness and a public health crisis that affects millions of people worldwide. It is one of the most common and dangerous forms of cancers, accounting for 1.3 million deaths annually (WHO, 2009). This type of cancer is particularly deadly because its cells are highly metastatic (i.e., spread) and can enter the blood and spread to form tumors in other parts of the lung, or in other organs, such as the liver and the brain (Solomon et al., 1996). Further, during the final part of the twentieth century, the global cancer burden increased by two-fold, and it is expected that this increase will continue at the same level between 2000 and 2020, and will triple by 2030 (WHO, 2008). Worldwide cancer mortality has been estimated to be as high as 12 million deaths in 2030 (WHO, 2009).

To improve the health of future generations, and acknowledging that not all smokers develop lung cancer, medical researchers have intensified their efforts to clarify the role of diet in lung cancer development. In this context, many researchers have explored whether there is a relationship between vitamin E intake and lung cancer risk. Vitamin E, a fat-soluble antioxidant, includes several tocopherol and tocotrienol derivates (Comitato et al., 2009). In most cases, antioxidants are important part of our diet; they can inhibit the oxidation of other molecules and protect cells from damage caused by free radicals (Solomon et al., 1996). Vitamin E, in particular, can deactivate free radicals, inhibit proliferation and induce apoptosis in a large number of cancer cells (Comitato et al., 2009); hence, it has the capacity to prevent some of the oxidative damage that may possibly cause (lung) cancer. As a result, diets rich in antioxidants, such as vitamin E, have been recommended to reduce the risk of developing cancers (Key et al., 2002). And yet, the dose-response effects of vitamin E intake on lung cancer risk and the molecular mechanism(s) involved in its action are still unclear.

This topic is relevant globally. According to WHO, there is evidence that effective cancer control measures will reduce the incidence of cancer significantly (WHO, 2008). Already in 2003, WHO argued that smoking cessation, healthy diet, and infection control would prevent as many as one third of cancers worldwide (WHO, 2003). Additionally, cancer has moved from being the disease of the wealthy in developed countries to becoming the disease of the poor in developing countries, where health care has traditionally been regarded as low priority (WHO, 2008). Health systems around the globe are facing severe challenges in terms of providing treatment to individuals suffering from cancers, including those of the lungs. In certain areas, limited funding prevents many cancer patients from receiving program benefits. This lack of funds may also prevent medical researchers from developing new treatments, and novel prevention approaches. All these factors have serious implications on society as a whole.

Nevertheless, despite the global and scientific relevance of the topic, human biological systems (in different parts of the world) are far from uniform, and it is not easy to determine whether the risk of developing lung cancer is reduced or increased by exposure to vitamin E during different phases of human life.

Book Highlights

This book explores different aspects of the dose-response relationship of vitamin E and lung cancer risk, focusing on assessing the empirical dose-response models of dietary and supplemental vitamin E intake on lung cancer risk and identified and proposed mechanism-based models. Although such an assessment may seem complicated and difficult at first, the book proposes a coherent, structured and progressive framework that can be useful not only when evaluating vitamin E intake, but also that of other micronutrients, macronutrients, or even toxic chemicals in relation to not only lung cancer, but also other types of cancer or chronic diseases.

Individual chapters emphasize, wherever possible, existing knowledge on biological processes (within the cells) that are capable of selectively inducing apoptosis of potential tumor cells. Thoughtful discussion is also given to the types of data available from research studies that have the potential to impact the development of dose-response models. Throughout the book, knowledge gaps relating to the evaluation of vitamin E dose-response are identified. This book highlights that, while significant achievements have been made in recent years, gaps in knowledge are still wide, and they constitute considerable constraints to the development of effective, novel and appropriately targeted (lung) cancer strategies. It is believed that understanding these gaps and their implications can guide the design of new dose-response studies that will add to our knowledge of vitamin E activity and shed light on issues related to its dose-response.

In particular, the book attempts to draw attention to the following questions:

- What does previous research reveal about whether dietary and supplemental intakes of vitamin E affect the risk of developing lung cancer?
- What is the shape of the dose-response curve for lung cancer risk at various doses of vitamin E?
- What is the safe or beneficial dose of vitamin E in relation to lung cancer risk?
- What is the critical dose at which no beneficial effects of vitamin E are observed?
- What are the empirical dose-response models and the mechanisms-based models of vitamin E that have been investigated previously with respect to lung cancer?

Chapter 1 (Dose Effects Of Vitamin E On Lung Cancer Risk)

The first chapter of the book generally emphasizes that the main advantage associated with conducting a dose-response analysis of vitamin E intake in relation to lung cancer risk is to detect and quantify the relationship between the dose of vitamin E and its effect on lung cancer development. This opening chapter outlines the broad principles of dose-response modeling and reviews very briefly some defining aspects of carcinogenesis in lung cancer, and the characteristics of dose effects of vitamin E on lung cancer risk.

Chapter 2 (Empirical Vitamin E-lung Cancer Risk Models)

The second chapter builds on these characteristics by assessing the strengths and weaknesses of two research studies, namely "Long-term use of supplemental multivitamins, vitamin C, vitamin E, and folate does not reduce the risk of lung cancer" by Slatore et al. (2008) and "Development of a Comprehensive Dietary Antioxidant Index and Application to Lung Cancer Risk in a Cohort of Male Smokers" by Wright et al. (2004). The main objective was to report on estimates of safe and critical dietary and supplemental doses of vitamin E consumption. Beneficial dietary and supplemental doses of vitamin E among Finish men aged 50-69 years who smoked five or more cigarettes per day and American men and women aged 50-76 years, respectively, are compared to their corresponding critical doses. An in-depth reflection on the methodology and data analysis employed by the researchers necessitated a focus on the complexity of the models presented, the interpretations that were made, and the uncertainties associated with not only the dose estimates of dietary and supplemental consumption of vitamin E, but also those associated with extrapolation of dose-response curves.

Chapter 3 (Mechanism-based Vitamin E-lung Cancer Models)

The third chapter presents several possible mechanisms and biological processes driving the development of lung cancer and connecting it to vitamin E status in serum or tissue. It provides detailed discussion on Fas signaling and transforming growth factor-beta pathways in a comprehensive literature review. It then goes on to discuss and, to a certain degree, evaluate the different modeling approaches. This chapter finds that the sphingomyelin signal transduction pathway and Rac1 pathway may be novel mechanism-based vitamin E-lung cancer models that have not yet been evaluated properly.

Chapter 4 (Conclusions And Implications)

The overall conclusions and implications are stated clearly in the final part. As the chapters in this book demonstrate, challenges involved in examining dose-response relationships of vitamin E and lung cancer risk can be recognized as some of the major barriers to developing and implementing a cohesive approach to lung cancer prevention, early detection, and treatment.

Before presenting each chapter, it is imperative to provide brief summaries of the two cohort studies that will be evaluated extensively in the present assessment.

Study One: The Vital Cohort

In the article "Long-Term Use of Supplemental Multivitamins, Vitamin C, Vitamin E, and Folate Does Not Reduce the Risk of Lung Cancer," which appeared in the American Journal of Respiratory and Critical Care Medicine in 2008, Christopher G. Slatore, Alyson J. Littman, David H. Au, Jessie A. Satia, and Emily White examined the association of supplemental multivitamins, vitamin E, vitamin C, and folate with the incidence of lung cancer (Slatore et al., 2008). Acknowledging the fact that lung cancer is the leading cause of cancer-related mortality in the United States, they explored data from a prospective cohort of 77,721 men and women aged 50-76 years from Washington State in the VITAL (VITamins And Lifestyle) study. Lung cancer cases were identified through the Seattle-Puget Sound SEER (Surveillance, Epidemiology, and End Results) cancer registry, which is reliable for lung cancer histology. Using a commercial list, 364,418 VITAL-supplement-questionnaires were mailed from October 2000-December 2002, and a total of 77,719 (21.3%) individuals who returned the questionnaires were identified as eligible subjects. Baseline data were collected, and the Institutional Review Board of the Fred Hutchinson Cancer Research Center approved the protocol.

Participants were monitored until 31 December 2005 by linking them to the Seattle-Puget Sound SEER registry. Mortality was ascertained through linkage to Washington State death files, while moves out of the area were obtained by linking the cohort to the National Change of Address System and by follow-up letters and telephone calls.

The covariates included in this study were tobacco, body mass index (BMI), socioeconomic and anthropomorphic factors, as well as previous history of cancer and self-report of physician-diagnosed chronic obstructive pulmonary disease (COPD) and/or asthma.

All statistical analyses were performed using Stata SE-9 (StataCorp, College Station, TX), and Cox regression was employed to estimate the hazard ratios (*HR*s) for associations of supplemental multivitamin, vitamin E, vitamin C, and folate use with lung cancer. To be more precise, the measurement was *HR*s for incident lung cancer according to 10-year average daily or weekly use of supplemental multivitamins, vitamin E, vitamin C, and folate.

Slatore and colleagues also examined the associations between different lung cancer morphologies and supplemental vitamins, as well as the differences of the supplement-lung cancer associations by subgroups defined by smoking status.

A total of 521 cases of lung cancer were identified. Adjusting for smoking, age, and gender, there was no inverse association with any supplement, whereas supplemental vitamin E was associated with a small increased risk of lung cancer (*HR*, 1.05 for every 100-mg/d increase in dose; 95% *CI* = 1.00-1.09; p = .033) (Slatore et al., 2008). The risk was greatest for non-small cell lung cancer (*HR*, 1.07 for every 100-mg/d increase; 95% *CI* = 1.02–1.12; p = .004) and was largely confined to current smokers (*HR*, 1.11 for every 100-mg/d increase; 95% *CI*,

1.03-1.19; $p = .01$). The study concluded that patients should be advised not to take vitamin E supplements to prevent lung cancer.

Study Two: The ATBC Cohort

The second article that is identified for critique and evaluation in this paper is entitled "Development of a Comprehensive Dietary Antioxidant Index and Application to Lung Cancer Risk in a Cohort of Male Smokers." Hypothesizing that multiple antioxidants simultaneously may be important in terms of risk estimation, Margaret E. Wright, Susan T. Mayne, Rachael Z. Stolzenberg-Solomon, Zhaohai Li, Pirjo Pietinen, Philip R. Taylor, Jarmo Virtamo, and Demetrius Albanes constructed a dietary antioxidant index and evaluated its ability to predict lung cancer risk within the Alpha-Tocopherol, Beta-Carotene (ATBC) Cancer Prevention Study cohort (Wright et al., 2004). The latter was a randomized, double-blinded, placebo-controlled primary chemoprevention trial with a 2×2 factorial design that tested whether supplementation with vitamin E (50 mg of dl-α-tocopherol/day) and β-carotene (20 mg/day) reduced the incidence of lung cancer (The ATBC Cancer Prevention Study Group, 1994).

At baseline (1985-1988), 27,111 Finnish males aged 50-69 years who smoked five or more cigarettes daily and were willing to provide written informed consent completed a dietary questionnaire that covered both food and beverages. Further, the institutional review boards of both the National Public Health

Institute of Finland, and the US National Cancer Institute approved the study. Incident primary cancers of the lung or bronchus were ascertained via the Finnish Cancer Registry, while administration of a chest radiograph at baseline ensured that men with apparent lung cancer were excluded from the trial. In addition, three follow-up chest radiographs were performed during the trial and at study exit. A total of 1,787 incident cases of lung cancer were identified during a follow-up period of up to 14.4 years (1985-1999, median, 11.3 years). Histologic verification was available for 95% of all cases.

Principal components analyses were individually applied to the vitamin E (α-tocopherol, γ-tocopherol, α-tocotrienol, and β-tocotrienol), carotenoid (α-carotene, β-carotene, β-cryptoxanthin, γ-carotene, lutein + zeaxanthin, and lycopene), and flavonoid (catechin, epicatechin, kaempferol, myricetin, and quercetin) nutrient groups, and summation of retained principal component scores, plus selenium and vitamin C, yielded the composite antioxidant index. These antioxidant nutrients were frequently consumed in this cohort.

The results indicated that, within each arm of the trial, risks of lung cancer were 13-18% lower among participants in the highest antioxidant index quintile compared with the lowest. Additionally, in multivariate proportional hazards models, the relative risks for lung cancer according to increasing quintiles of the antioxidant index were 1.00 (referent), 1.00 (95% *CI*: 0.87, 1.14), 0.91 (95% *CI*: 0.79, 1.05), 0.79 (95% *CI*: 0.68, 0.92), and 0.84 (95% *CI*: 0.72, 0.98) (p for trend = .002).

Accordingly, Wright et al. (2004) concluded that their findings supported the hypothesis that a combination of dietary antioxidants reduced lung cancer risk in male smokers. Thus, a balanced diet rich in a variety of antioxidant nutrients was recommended because it may play an important role in the fight against lung cancer in smokers. The researchers stated, however, that the benefits appeared to be modest and that the fundamental strategy in the prevention of lung cancer should still be smoking cessation.

CHAPTER 1: DOSE EFFECTS OF VITAMIN E ON LUNG CANCER RISK

Abstract

This chapter outlines the characteristics of dose-response relationships of lung cancer responses induced by various doses and sources of vitamin E. Whether or not knowledge of possible molecular mechanisms connecting vitamin E intake to lung cancer risk is helpful for the evaluation of dose-response models is also addressed. Admittedly, some of the targeted aspects may be difficult to address and therefore they have too often been overlooked in previous analyses, but are too important to be passed over. It is accepted by most investigators that most cellular responses to vitamin E require the initial interaction between vitamin E and the Fas Ligand and/or the inactive (latent) transforming growth factor-beta (TGF-β). Many of the biological responses to certain vitamin E compounds at the cellular level appear to depend on the induction of apoptosis in pulmonary epithelium and lymphoid cells. However, it must be kept in mind that the dose-response characteristics of vitamin E action are believed to be strengthened by additional mechanistic pathways that are yet to be identified.

Characteristics of Dose Effect of Vitamin E on Lung Cancer Risk

A dose-response relationship describes how the likelihood and severity of adverse health effects (i.e., the responses) are related to the different levels (i.e., the doses) of exposure to the factor of interest after a certain exposure time (U.S. EPA, n.d.). The shape of the dose-response relationship depends on the type of response (e.g., lung cancer risk, incidence of lung cancer, mortality) that is observed, the dose given that produced that response, and the subjects (e.g., humans, animals, or isolated lung cells or tissue) tested. For instance, the relationship observed for a response like "lung cancer risk" maybe different from the relationship observed for a response like "lung cancer mortality" or "lung cancer incidence." Besides, use of vitamin E supplements over an extended period of time (over 8 years) may increase the risk of developing lung cancer among American men and women aged 50-76 years (Slatore et al., 2008), whereas supplementing with small amounts of vitamin E may produce no observable effect in the same population or in other populations. To put it differently, different populations may respond differently at different doses and exposure times.

There are many advantages associated with conducting a dose-response analysis of the effects of vitamin E intake on lung cancer risk. The main advantage is that a dose-response analysis detects and quantifies the relationship between a dose of the exposure under consideration and its effect on human health, i.e., in the present context, an increasing intake of vitamin E and its effect on lung cancer development. Other advantages include making comparisons between the various forms of vitamin E across a wide dose range, and even with limited data, certain forms of vitamin E with similar mechanism of actions may have a similar shape or similar maximal effect (Mandema et al., 2005). Most importantly, the most compelling evidence of causality in epidemiological studies is the presence of a dose-response relationship (NAS, 1995). That is, the demonstration of a trend in the lung cancer risk (or incidence) with degree or duration of vitamin E intake.

In relation to this analysis, two major elements can be distinguished: Dose and response. On the one hand, examples of dose include the amount of supplemental and dietary vitamin E taken by, for instance, cohort members at a given frequency. In other words, the magnitude of lung cancer risk that is caused by vitamin E exposure depends on the dose and frequency of vitamin E intake. The extent and magnitude of the effects of vitamin E are mediated through its ability to activate certain cell surface receptors (see *Mechanism-Based Vitamin E-Lung Cancer Models* in Chapter 3). This stimulation results in a sequence of biochemical events that are linked to particular biological functions, including cell cycle arrest and apoptosis, each of which may reflect simple (or light) responses with a low and time-limited exposure or complicated responses with high and prolonged exposure.

It is worthwhile here to emphasize that two of the biochemical effects of vitamin E that might have particular relevance to its protective effects are (a) its ability to inhibit cancer formation by quenching of free radicals; and (b) its control of tumor growth through the induction of differentiation and apoptosis (Kline et al., 2001). Additionally, although desired, the actual dose that cause a specific response (i.e., the activation of a specific mechanism of action) remains unknown, and the best estimates reported in this book are based on a number of assumptions and parameters presented in previous studies. The more well-designed the study is (i.e., the higher the precision and validity of the study), the closer the estimates are to the actual dose (i.e., the more confident the researcher would be in the obtained estimates).

On the other hand, a response can be regarded as an observation or a result following exposure to vitamin E. Responses may include a wide spectrum of observations or outcomes, from simple biochemical reactions to complex events, some of which are tissue-specific and may be directly or indirectly, positively or inversely related to exposure dose. In this regard, research has demonstrated that cancer is caused by mutations in the DNA, and that carcinogens in tobacco smoke may trigger mutations in lung cells, leading in certain cases to lung cancer; thus, the causes of mutations in lung cells are believed to be the causes of lung cancer (MedlinePlus, 2013). However, one of the major challenges that face researchers is to figure out the biological pathways that start with genetic mutations and may result in a response like lung cancer.

At the same time, research has revealed that vitamin E succinate (VES), i.e., the succinated form of *RRR*- α-tocopherol that is often used in vitamin E supplements, is a potent inducer of apoptosis in a wide range of human cancer cells and have been found to effectively *induce apoptosis in a dose* and time dependant manner (Kline et al., 2001). For instance, this derivative of vitamin E at a 50% effective concentration range of 5-10 mg/L is capable of inducing human lung (A549) cells to undergo apoptosis (Kline et al., 2001).

An overall hypothesis for the mode of action of vitamin E, put forth by a number of researchers, is based on different pathways, many of which are related to the inhibition and/or activation of the expression of certain genes. This hypothesis has been most well characterized for the identification of SMAD3 as a repressor of human telomerase reverse transcriptase (*hTERT*) gene and the *c-myc* gene, i.e., the gene that contributes to the development of human cancers (Li et al., 2006). There is also some evidence indicating that the activation of p53 transcription factor is impaired in 55% of lung cancer patients who are smokers, compared to 38% of lung cancer patients who are former smokers (had stopped smoking 1-5 years earlier), and 25% of those who are nonsmokers (Husgafvel-Pursiainen & Kannio, 1996). The biological basis for these findings and their possible influence on suggested pathways is outlined in the following chapters.

Although gaps in knowledge still exist, research to date is consistent with the hypothesis that treatment with VES induces apoptosis in human cancer cells by converting latent inactive transforming growth factor-beta (TGF-β) to its active form and/or up-regulating the expression of Fas ligand, both of which represent the first steps in a series of biochemical and cellular changes that may define the benefits observed (Kline at al., 2001). The evidence that supports this theory has been presented in chapter 3 after conducting a comprehensive literature review (e.g., Pearson et al., 2001; Kline et al., 2001; Wajant, 2002; Takayama et al., 2001; Bignold, 2004; Sterner-Kock et al., Ishisaki et al., 1999; Wharton & Derynck, 2009; Hariharan & Pillai, 2008).

Finally, many of the known biological activities of tocopherols and tocotrienols also appear to follow their rank order of activating other apoptotic pathways, such as sphingomyelin signal transduction pathway and Rac1-induced apoptosis pathway (see chapter 3). The sphingomyelin pathway mediates apoptosis in several nonhematopoietic cells and holds for changes in concentration of several proteins, including the generation of ceramides, which leads to DNA fragmentation in sensitive cells (Haimovitz-Friedman, 1994). The direct relationship between vitamin E and the generation of ceramides is less clear. But although evidence are limited, it can be hypothesized that many of the biochemical effects produced by vitamin E in Fas signaling and TGF-β signaling pathways may also occur in sphingomyelin signal transduction pathway and Rac1-induced apoptosis. This hypothesis is novel because as of yet (a) only one study has revealed that a combination of vitamin E forms induces cell death in human prostate cancer cells by interrupting sphingolipid synthesis (Jiang et al., 2004); and to date (b) almost no studies have examined Rac1-induced apoptosis as a possible mechanism of action for vitamin E in relation to lung cancer risk.

Dose-Response Modeling

Dose response modeling involves the development of computational (mathematical) systems and biological tools to predict and understand the dose-response relationship for certain components (e.g., combinations of vitamin E forms) at the cellular and tissue level of the target organ (i.e., human lung) (Zhang, n.d.). Such models are generally classified as either empirical models or mechanism-based models (Hoel, 1980). Both categories are briefly reviewed in the next chapters.

In this respect, human dose-response testing is based on epidemiological data that compares "exposed" to "unexposed" individuals. However, the "unexposed" study subjects may contain substantial amounts of background exposure to antioxidants, including vitamin E, in the absence or presence of other identified and unidentified risk factors. Also, the results of many epidemiological studies are hampered by small sample sizes, and in most cases, the actual amounts of vitamin E in human tissues are not examined. It is not often either that serum vitamin E levels are measured. In addition, in populations exposed to similar amounts of vitamin E (e.g., the population examined in Wright et al. study), some subjects may exhibit a reduced risk of lung cancer while others may not. This suggests that there may be multiple factors (e.g., genetic susceptibility, radon exposure) that may influence an individual's response to the dose of vitamin E consumed. Consequently, the concept of independent versus additive backgrounds must be taken into consideration (Hoel, 1980). Additive background implies linearity, while the assumption of total independence of background is necessary to justify nonlinearity at low doses (Hoel, 1980). This aspect has important implications to low-dose extrapolations for the purpose of risk estimation.

Dose-response models for ligand-receptor mediated pathways are supposed to use information on key associations between ligand-activated receptors and biological response. It should be noted here that at very low concentrations of vitamin E, the receptor occupancy of TGF-β and/or Fas receptor may occur, but it may not be enough to induce apoptosis. On the other hand, if there are a sufficient number of receptors per cell, the number of death-inducing signaling complexes formed can be significant even at low vitamin E levels. One advantage of this approach is that the mechanism of action of the exposure of interest (in this case vitamin E intake) is considered sensitive to changes in exposure concentration (i.e., the levels of vitamin E intake that reflect the levels of vitamin E in tissues) (Roth & Grunfield, 1985).

Clearly, multiple dose-response models can be employed when dealing with ligand-receptor mediated pathways. More specifically, when there is a proportional relationship between receptor occupancy and biological response, occupancy of any number of receptors, such as type II and type I Serine-Threonine Kinases (STKs) (see chapter 3), would produce a response; however, the response is more likely to be detectable only if an adequate number of receptors are activated simultaneously. Thus, if the number of receptors occupied is very low, a simple model that describes the response as a linear function of dose will probably be appropriate. Nonetheless, such a simple model is inadequate to provide a complete picture of the complexity and diversity of the biological responses that are initiated by a single receptor that is receptive to vitamin E effects.

That said, the dose-response relationships for relatively simple responses (e.g., the translocation of DAXX from the nucleus to the cytoplasm; see chapter 3) are unlikely to be used to analyze and/or predict the dose-response relationships for complex responses, such as lung cancer development. As a result, it is imperative to take into account what is known and hypothesized about the biological responses before analyzing the mathematical models applied to the data at hand in the two reviewed studies.

CHAPTER 2: EMPIRICAL MODELS OF VITAMIN E-LUNG CANCER RISK

Abstract

The dose-response relationship between vitamin E intake and lung cancer risk has been examined in some studies; however the evidence is inconclusive. In this chapter, using data from two selected cohort studies, the dose-response relationships between dietary and supplemental intakes of vitamin E and lung cancer risk were assessed. The results of this assessment suggested that the estimated safe and beneficial dietary dose of vitamin E among Finish male smokers (five or more cigarettes per day) aged 50-69 years was 15-26.74 mg per day, while the estimated critical dose was 30.06 mg per day. Furthermore, the estimated safe dose of supplemental vitamin E among American men and women aged 50-76 years was 42-215 mg per day, whereas the estimated critical dose was greater than 215 mg per day. Overall, whereas smoking cessation is believed to reduce the risk of developing lung cancer, sufficient levels of vitamin E intake (15 mg/day), including daily consumption of fruits and vegetables, may provide a key dietary strategy in lung cancer prevention. Given the limitations and potential biases inherent in cohort studies, the estimated doses need to be confirmed in further investigations.

Empirical Dose-Response Models

At the beginning of this section, it is important to highlight that data applicable to empirical dose-response modeling can usually be expressed through groups of subjects exposed to a certain level of vitamin E for which some response is determined. Given the research studies conducted in recent years, it is likely that a pattern will emerge, which can be applied to assess the change in the response as a function of increased or decreased dose. The main goal of *empirical dose-response modeling* is to construct a simple mathematical model that adequately describes the pattern of the dose-response relationship (Bonamin, 2008). Although these models often do not consider the underlying mechanisms that drive a specific response, they are usually interpreted in light of the knowledge available with respect to the biological responses considered, thereby providing a better assessment of the underlying mechanisms (Bonamin, 2008). Examples of empirical models include, but are not limited to, (a) linear functions; (b) log-linear models; (c) poisson regression that are commonly used in epidemiology; and most importantly (d) Hill models that are commonly used to analyze ligand-receptor data (Bonamin, 2008).

Dose-Response Models On Vitamin E Intake To Lung Cancer Risk

The modeling approaches used in the studies presented in this book involves applying estimated lung cancer response and estimating the hazard ratios or relative risks for each data set. In both studies, Cox regression models were used to examine the effects of supplemental or dietary vitamin E and the studied covariates on the risk of developing lung cancer. In the study conducted by Slatore et al. (2008), there were three exposure groups and one reference group, whereas there were five groups in the study conducted by Wright et al. (2004), of which the first one was considered a reference group.

Obviously, with this kind of data, the researchers could have used other empirical dose-response models. Alternatively, they could have applied the probabilistic Hill equation, which permits the estimation of the probability of an adverse event of a given daily dosage of vitamin E. Although the Hill equation is often used in models of gene regulation, its many advantages and potential applications in pharmacology and biosciences are not all well known (Goutelle et al., 2008). This approach could be a powerful tool to analyze quantitative vitamin E-receptor relationships to evaluate and to choose the most appropriate dose of vitamin E, taking into account both the expected benefits and potential toxicity of vitamin E (Goutelle et al., 2008).

And yet, having in mind the complexity of cohort data, the influence of uncontrolled confounding variables, the degree of bias in the data, and the variation in the accuracy and precision of exposure estimates, the application of the broadly used Cox models seem adequate. These are the most general types of regression models because they are not based on any assumptions about the nature or shape of the underlying survival distribution (StatSoft, 2010). The main advantage of using Cox regression models is that they are capable of handling the time-dependent covariates, such as changing smoking habits throughout the study (Allison, *2003*). Such models assume that the underlying hazard rate is a function of the independent variable(s) (or the covariates or potential predictors); thus, in a sense, Cox regression models can be considered as a nonparametric method (StatSoft, 2010). The model can be described by the following formula:

$$\mathbf{H(t) = H_0(t) * exp(\beta_1 X_1 + ... + \beta_m X_m)}$$

where $H(t)$ denotes the probability of the endpoint (lung cancer), $H_0(t)$ is the baseline hazard (i.e., the hazard for an individual when all values of possible predictor variables are equal to zero), given the values of the *m* covariates for the respective predictor variables (X_1, ..., X_m) and the respective survival time *(t)* (StatSoft, 2010; MedCalc, 2011). In order to linearize this model (i.e., to construct a simple linear model that concisely can describe the results of a study), both sides of the equation can be divided by $H_0(t)$ and then by taking the natural logarithm of both sides yields (StatSoft, 2010; MedCalc, 2011):

$$\mathbf{ln\ [H(t)/H_0(t)] = \beta_1 X_1 + ... + \beta_m X_m}$$

where $H(t)/H_0(t)$ is the hazard ratio. The coefficients $\beta_1 ... \beta_m$ are estimated by Cox regression. From this equation, it appears that the quantity $e^{\beta i}$ can be interpreted as the instantaneous relative risk of lung cancer development at any time for an individual with the risk factor present (e.g., a person who eats insufficient amounts of vitamin E or toxic amounts of vitamin E) compared with an individual with the risk factor absent (i.e., a person who eats adequate amounts of vitamin E), provided that both individuals are the same on all other covariates, i.e., if the ceteris paribus assumption is adequately satisfied.Although no assumptions are made about the shape of the underlying hazard function, the presented equations above define the two assumptions that should be taken into account. The first assumption is the proportionality assumption, which states that there is a multiplicative relationship between the underlying hazard function and the log-linear function of the covariates (Cox, 1972). The second assumption is that there is a log-linear relationship between the independent variables and the underlying hazard function (Statistical Solutions, n.d.).Before presenting the results of Cox models, it must be noted that, due to the lack of access to the raw data, no comprehensive assessment of the shape of the dose-response relationships was conducted.

The VITAL Cohort

In the VITAL cohort, Slatore et al. (2008) analyzed long-term intensity of vitamin E supplement intake using data from a cohort of 77,721 men and women aged 50-76 years from Washington State, considering only lung cancers occurring after 10 years of exposure. The participants were classified into groups by the average daily use of supplemental vitamin E and the average weekly use of supplemental multivitamins: No vitamin E use, 1st tertile <42 mg/d, 2nd tertile = 42-215 mg/d, and 3rd tertile >215 mg/d, versus no multivitamin use, 1st tertile >0-

2.8 pills/wk, 2nd tertile >2.8-5.6 pills/wk, and 3rd tertile >5.6 pills/wk. As mentioned earlier, this study included a dose-response analysis by a Cox regression model, which calculated the hazard ratios for lung cancer associated with 10-year use of supplemental vitamin E and supplemental multivitamins, with cigarette smoking, BMI, previous history of cancer, self-report of physician-diagnosed chronic obstructive pulmonary disease (COPD), and socioeconomic and anthropomorphic factors included as explanatory variables. To be more precise, the model that was used is the Cox's proportional hazard model with time-dependent covariates, which allows analyzing the effect of several risk factors on survival (MedCalc, 2011). By simplifying and using the Cox equation mentioned earlier, the hazard ratio for a 10-year use of supplemental vitamin E would be as follows:

$$\mathbf{HR}_{\textbf{lung cancer/10-year use of supplemental vitamin E}} = \mathbf{e}^{\boldsymbol{\beta}\textbf{vitaminE(10)}}$$

The findings of the reviewed study are reported in Table 1 and Table 2. The long-term use of supplemental vitamin E was found to be significantly associated with a small increased risk of lung cancer ($HR = 1.05$ for every 100-mg/d increase in dose; 95% CI: 1.00-1.09; $p = .033$), which was most prominent in current smokers ($HR = 1.11$ for every 100-mg/d increase; 95% CI: 1.03–1.19; $p < .01$) and for non-small cell lung cancer ($HR = 1.07$ for every 100-mg/d increase; 95% CI: 1.02–1.12; $p = .004$) (Slatore et al., 2008). The findings also indicated a possible U-shaped association, i.e., subjects using a medium dose of supplemental vitamin E for 10 years had a decreased risk of lung cancer, whereas those using a high dose for 10 years showed an increased risk (Slatore et al., 2008).

Moreover, Table 3 and Table 4 summarize the results of the association of supplemental vitamin E and multivitamin use stratified by smoking status. As seen in Table 3, there was no significant association between incident lung cancer and supplemental multivitamin use neither for current nor for former smokers. In contrast, the results in Table 4 showed an increased risk of developing lung cancer for every 100-mg/day increase in supplemental vitamin E (HR = 1.11; 95% CI: 1.03-1.19; $p < .01$) for current smokers, with an overall p value for interaction of .06 (Slatore et al., 2008). Current smokers in the highest dose category had a significantly increased risk of lung cancer (HR = 1.59; 95% CI: 1.05-2.41; p for trend $< .01$), whereas there was no significant association between incident lung cancer and supplemental vitamin E for either group of former smokers (see Table 4 below) (Slatore et al., 2008).

Evidently, the hazard ratio can verify whether the probability of lung cancer development is the same among exposure groups. In this case, as long as the hazard ratio is greater than 1, a hazard exists. In other words, there is an association between supplemental vitamin E use and survival experience related to lung cancer.

Table 1. *Hazard Ratios for Lung Cancer Associated with 10-year Use of Supplemental Vitamin E in the Prospective Cohort of 77,721 Men and Women Aged 50-76 Years from Washington State in the VITAL Study* (Slatore *et al., 2008)*

Vitamin use	Non-cases *N* = 76,605	Cases *N* = 521	Adjusted Hazard Ratio (95% *CI*)
No Vitamin E use	19,963 (26.3)	146 (28.4)	1.0 Reference
1st tertile: <42 mg/d	18,676 (24.6)	115 (22.3)	0.97 (0.76-1.25)
2nd tertile: 42–215 mg/d	18,604 (24.5)	93 (18.1)	0.80 (0.62-1.04)
3rd tertile: >215 mg/d	18,778 (24.7)	161 (31.3)	1.19 (0.95-1.50)

Note: Values for non-cases and cases are number (%). All supplements had <5% missing data and percentages are of total; numbers may not sum to 100% secondary to missing data and/or rounding. p trend = .03. Hazard ratio = 1.05 for every 100 mg/day. Values are adjusted for age, gender, years smoked, pack-years, and pack-years squared.

Table 2. *Hazard Ratios for Lung Cancer Associated with 10-year Use of Supplemental Multivitamins in the Prospective Cohort of 77,721 Men and Women Aged 50-76 Years from Washington State in the VITAL Study* (Slatore *et al., 2008)*

Vitamin use	Non-cases *N* = 76,605	Cases *N* = 521	Adjusted Hazard Ratio (95% *CI*)
No Multivitamin use	26,440 (34.5)	183 (35.1)	1.0 Reference
1st tertile: >0-2.8 pills/wk	15,912 (20.8)	106 (20.4)	1.21 (0.95-1.54)
2nd tertile: >2.8-5.6 pills/wk	14,602 (19.1)	90 (17.3)	1.08 (0.84-1.39)
3rd tertile: >5.6 pills/wk	19,641 (25.6)	142 (27.3)	0.98 (0.78-1.22)

Note: Values for non-cases and cases are number (%). All supplements had <5% missing data and percentages are of total; numbers may not sum to 100% secondary to missing data and/or rounding. *p* trend = .69. Values are adjusted for age, gender, years smoked, pack-years, and pack-years squared.

Table 3. *Hazard Ratios for Lung Cancer Associated with 10-year Use of Supplemental Multivitamins Stratified by Smoking Status in the Prospective Cohort of 77,721 Men and Women Aged 50-76 Years from Washington State in the VITAL Study* (Slatore *et al., 2008)*

	Adjusted Hazard Ratio (95% *CI*)		
Vitamin use	Current smokers	Former smokers quit < 10yr	Former smokers quit ≥10yr
No multivitamin use	1.00 Reference	1.00 Reference	1.00 Reference
1st tertile: >0-2.8 pills/wk	1.12 (0.72-1.73)	1.29 (0.76-2.17)	1.16 (0.80-1.68)
2nd tertile: >2.8-5.6 pills/wk	1.23 (0.77-1.94)	0.94 (0.52-1.72)	0.91 (0.62-1.35)
3rd tertile: >5.6 pills/wk	1.02 (0.67-1.56)	0.70 (0.39-1.25)	0.96 (0.69-1.32)
--	*p* trend = .76	*p* trend = .16	*P* trend = .60

Note: Values are adjusted for age, gender, years smoked, pack-years, and pack-years squared. *p* for interaction = .41.

Table 4. *Hazard Ratios for Lung Cancer Associated with 10-year Use of Supplemental Vitamin E Stratified by Smoking Status in the Prospective Cohort of 77,721 Men and Women Aged 50-76 Years from Washington State in the VITAL Study (*Slatore *et al., 2008)*

	Adjusted Hazard Ratio (95% *CI*)		
Vitamin use	Current smokers	Former smokers quit < 10yr	Former smokers quit ≥10yr
No Vitamin E use	1.00 Reference	1.00 Reference	1.00 Reference
1st tertile: <42 mg/d	1.06 (0.69-1.63)	0.72 (0.41-1.27)	0.90 (0.61-1.33)
2nd tertile: 42–215 mg/d	0.68 (0.40-1.18)	0.80 (0.46-1.40)	0.86 (0.58-1.26)
3rd tertile: >215 mg/d	1.59 (1.05-2.41)	0.77 (0.44-1.36)	1.11 (0.79-1.57)
--	p trend < .01	p trend = .28	P trend = .26

Note: Values are adjusted for age, gender, years smoked, pack-years, and pack-years squared. Hazard ratio = 1.11 for every 100-mg/day increase. p for interaction = .06.

In evaluating these results, the significant evidence of an increased lung cancer risk at a particular dose of supplemental vitamin E may alert the observers to the possibility that cohort subjects have been subjected to exposures that have increased their risk of developing lung cancer. Still, a single elevated hazard ratio is not always considered as a strong evidence for a causal association, unless its magnitude exceeds any value that can be justified in terms of logical reasoning, previous research, or potential experimental biases.

The ATBC Cohort

Another cohort study evaluated in this paper consisted of 27,111 Finnish men aged 50-69 years who smoked five or more cigarettes per day (Wright et al., 2004). An antioxidant index that included the consumption of vitamin E, caroteniods and flavonoids was used to express the relative antioxidant effect on lung cancer risk. Pearson correlation coefficients within nutrient groups ranged from 0.007 to 0.85 for the vitamin E, from 0.17 to 0.99 for the carotenoids, and from 0.61 to 0.99 for the flavonoids isomers (Wright et al., 2004). For a given set of nutrients, each principal component was computed by first multiplying the standardized intake of a specific nutrient by its corresponding weight, or factor loading, and subsequently summing across all contributing nutrients to obtain a score for each study participant. The first principal component within each nutrient group accounted for the largest proportion of the total variance in intake (vitamin E: 59%; carotenoids: 54%; flavonoids: 81%) and was retained for further analysis (Wright et al., 2004).

The index was divided into quintiles based on the distribution in the entire cohort, and Cox regression was used to calculate the relative risks for lung cancer. The analyses were stratified by intervention assignment (α-tocopherol, no α-tocopherol, β-carotene, no β-carotene), smoking intensity (cigarettes/day), histologic type (squamous cell carcinoma, small cell carcinoma, adenocarcinoma, other carcinoma), stage of disease (tumor-node-metastasis stages I-IV), alcohol consumption (0, > 0 - ≤ 7.4, > 7.4 - ≤ 22.9, or > 22.9 g/day), age (≤ 57 years vs. > 57 years), and BMI (≤ 25 vs. > 25) to evaluate potential effect modification. The researchers also evaluated whether intake of the two most common putative pro-oxidant nutrients, polyunsaturated fatty acids derived from fish and heme iron, modified the association between the antioxidant index and lung cancer risk. Because information on heme iron was not available in the Finnish nutrient database, its consumption was estimated using previously published information on the heme iron contents of cooked poultry, beef, veal, pork, and frankfurters (Wright et al., 2004).

The researchers have chosen to look at vitamin E use as an independent predictor (i.e., yes/no use at baseline) of lung cancer incidence (Allison, *2003*). A test for trend of the relative risks with increasing vitamin E intake was conducted. In the calculations, the trend test was significant at $p < .01$ and .07 for *α-tocopherol* group and *no α-tocopherol* group, respectively. The results of this study for the association between α-tocopherol and lung cancer risk, stratified by trial intervention group, are presented in Table 5. It appears that risks of lung cancer were 13-18% lower among participants in the highest α-tocopherol quintile compared with the lowest, and the data disclosed no evidence of heterogeneity in these risk estimates (*p* for interaction = .99) (Wright et al., 2004). Additionally, in multivariate proportional hazards models, the relative risks for lung cancer according to increasing quintiles of α-tocopherol were 1.00 (referent), 0.98 (95% *CI*: 0.81-1.19), 0.86 (95% *CI*: 0.70-1.05), 0.77 (95% *CI*: 0.63-0.95), and 0.82

(95% *CI*: 0.66-1.01) (*p* for trend = .01). The inverse relation between the index and lung cancer was strongest among participants in the upper quartiles of heme iron intake, whereas it was not apparent among men in the lower quartiles of heme iron intake.

The experts highlighted, however, that they cannot be certain that the observed association between the antioxidant index and lung cancer risk was due to the antioxidant activity of the aforementioned nutrient groups. For instance, α-tocopherol and γ-tocopherol possess anti-proliferative and anti-inflammatory properties, respectively, which are independent of their antioxidant activities (Wright et al., 2004). Despite this, as the study showed that a combination of dietary antioxidants was more strongly protective against lung cancer among males consuming higher quantities of heme iron suggested that the index was in fact capturing antioxidant activity (Wright et al., 2004).

Table 5. *Multivariate Relative Risk* of Lung Cancer According to Quintile of α-Tocopherol, Stratified by Trial Intervention Arm, in the Alpha-Tocopherol, Beta-Carotene Cancer Prevention Study cohort, 1985-1999 (Wright et al., 2008)*

Quintile of α-tocopherol	α-tocopherol			No α-tocopherol		
	N	*RR*	95% *CI*	*N*	*RR*	95% *CI*
1st quintile	233	1.0		222	1.0	
2nd quintile	199	0.98	0.81-1.19	210	1.01	0.84-1.22
3rd quintile	172	0.86	0.70-1.05	174	0.97	0.80, 1.19
4th quintile	151	0.77	0.63-0.95	142	0.82	0.66, 1.02
5th quintile	145	0.82	0.66-1.01	139	0.87	0.70, 1.08
p for trend			.01			.07

* Adjusted for energy intake, age, number of cigarettes smoked per day, number of years of smoking, body mass index, and educational level. RR, relative risk; CI, confidence interval.

Interpretation Of Doses

Based on the results presented above, the safe versus critical levels (or doses) of vitamin E intake can be identified (see Table 6). The estimated safe and/or beneficial dose of supplemental vitamin E in the study conducted by Slatore et al. (2008) appeared to be 42 - 215 mg per day, which was equivalent to a hazard ratio for lung cancer associated with 10-year use of supplemental vitamin E of 0.80 (95% *CI*: 0.62-1.04, p trend = .03). Nonetheless, when the dose of supplemental vitamin E was greater than 215 mg per day, the hazard ratio for lung cancer associated with 10-year use of supplemental vitamin E increased and reached 1.19 (95% *CI*: 0.95-1.50, p trend = .03), presenting a percentage difference of 32.7%. In the current smoker group, the estimated critical dose of supplemental Vitamin E was found also to be greater than 215 mg per day, which showed a hazard ratio for lung cancer associated with 10-year use of supplemental vitamin E of 1.59 (95% CI: 1.05-2.41, p trend $< .01$, p for interaction = .06). Therefore, it is reasonable to conclude that the estimated critical dose of supplemental vitamin E use is > 215 mg per day.

Table 6. *The Safe versus Critical Doses of Supplemental Vitamin E Use versus Dietary Vitamin E Use in the VITAL (*Slatore *et al., 2008) and ATBC (Wright et al., 2008) Studies*

Vitamin E intake	Safe dose	Critical dose
Supplemental	42 - 215 mg/d	> 215 mg/d
Dietary	15 - 26.74 mg/d	30.06 mg/d

These results are consistent with the findings of the study conducted by Wright et al. (2004). Although Wright and colleagues had concluded that the relative risk of lung cancer reduces with increasing dose of α-tocopherol, *RR* = 1.00 (referent), 0.98 (95% *CI*: 0.81-1.19), 0.86 (95% *CI*: 0.70-1.05), 0.77 (95% *CI*: 0.63-0.95), and 0.82 (95% *CI*: 0.66-1.01), *p* for trend = .01, a closer inspection of the results reveals that the relative risk of lung cancer was decreasing with increasing dose of α-tocopherol until it reached 0.77 in the 4th quintile (α-tocopherol = 11.8 mg/d); however, it then increased again and became 0.82 in the 5th quintile (α-tocopherol = 13.4 mg/d).

In order to be able to interpret these findings on a sound basis, it is important to provide more detail on the recommended dietary allowance of vitamin E for adults. According to the Dietary Reference Intakes of the Institute of Medicine, adults over 18 years need 15 *mg of vitamin E daily* (DRIs, 2004). Therefore, a daily intake of naturally occurring vitamin E of at least 15 mg is considered adequate level of vitamin E, whereas doses less than 15 mg a day are considered low levels of dietary vitamin E intake.

Keeping these figures in mind, and also the baseline characteristics in Wright et al. (2004) study, it must be stated that the overall amount of vitamin E consumed by the participants did not only consist of α-tocopherol. In addition to other antioxidants and α-tocopherol, the subjects' dietary characteristics included intake of γ-tocopherol, α-tocotrienol, and β-tocotrienol. In other words, the subjects' intake of dietary vitamin E was as high as 30.06 mg per day in the 5th quintile, whereas the subjects' intake of dietary vitamin E was 15 to 26.74 mg per day in the 1st and 4th quintile, respectively. Thus, these figures imply that the estimated safe level of dietary vitamin E intake among male smokers in this study was 15-26.74 mg per day, while the estimated critical level of dietary intake of vitamin E was 30.06 mg per day (see Table 6 above).

In brief, this analysis suggested that the estimated safe dietary dose of vitamin E among Finish male smokers was 15-26.74 mg per day, while the estimated critical dose was 30.06 mg per day. Furthermore, the estimated safe and beneficial dose of supplemental vitamin E among American men and women was 42-215 mg per day, whereas the estimated critical dose was greater than 215 mg per day.

Uncertainties In Estimates

There are many uncertainties associated with risk estimates derived from epidemiological studies, both in hazard identification and in dose estimation. Estimates of dose were, for instance, based on questionnaires and may therefore not be fully precise or reliable. For example, although 77,721 men and women aged 50-76 years were sampled in the VITAL study, the data obtained were primarily based on the VITAL-supplement-questionnaires (Slatore et al., 2008), which can be affected by self-reporting bias.

Another element of uncertainty is related to the fact that variables can be closely connected and may somehow affect one another. In other words, it is essential to consider the extent to which any change in vitamin E use may influence the effects that smoking, BMI, and other variables may have on lung cancer risk. Therefore, the most important point to evaluate prior to conducting this kind of research is to evaluate how connected the variables are to each other.

A third source of uncertainty is related to the shape of the dose-response relationship. The tables reported earlier in this chapter showed, in general terms, a pattern of reducing the relative risks for lung cancer in male smokers with increasing dose of the antioxidant index in the ATBC Cancer Prevention Study cohort (Wright et al., 2004). In contrast, the VITAL cohort study found a pattern of reducing the adjusted hazard ratios for lung cancer associated with 10-year use of supplemental vitamin E in both sexes with increasing dose, but the adjusted hazard ratios for lung cancer then increased with increased vitamin E levels (Slatore et al., 2008). Thus, the latter dose-response model was not linear, but rather U-shaped.

When interpreting the risk estimates presented in this chapter, other potential biases and limitations must also be acknowledged. Both relative risks and hazard risks are attributed to vitamin E intake, even in the case of consuming other micronutrients. Specifically, although these analyses included the use of other antioxidants, the extent to which these micronutrients affected the findings discussed in this chapter (i.e., the various effects of these micronutrients on calculating the risk estimates of vitamin E) remains largely unknown. In other words, these confounders raise the question of whether the observed beneficial effects of vitamin E are attributed to vitamin E, uncontrolled confounding factors, or both.

Additionally, selection bias may be another issue of concern. For instance, it is possible that the subpopulations used for risk estimation who returned the questionnaires were not representative of the entire cohorts. Information bias, interviewer bias and reporting bias may have also occurred. There is also a potential bias due to the healthy lifestyle habits adopted by participants who had taken ownership of their health.

Discussion

Vitamin E intake can generate various responses depending on the dose-response relationship of the vitamin E use and the exposure scenario. The ATBC cancer prevention study clearly suggested a dietary vitamin E-mediated decrease in lung cancer, while the VITAL cohort demonstrated that supplemental vitamin E was associated with a small increased risk of lung cancer. Smoking and other confounding variables discussed above may act as modifiers for the development of lung cancer. In addition, the two studies under consideration here were designed to explore an observed effect of dietary intake or intake of supplementary antioxidants on lung cancer risk and, as such, these sets of data are supposed to contain sufficient dose-response information. Despite this, the results achieved cannot be considered conclusive. Besides, the hazard ratios and relative risks presented in Tables 1-5 are based on Cox proportional hazard models, in which the hazard ratio is assumed to be constant over time (Bewick et al., 2004). As a result, the use of untransformed survival times may make these models less appealing (Statistical Solutions, n.d.), and therefore, care must be taken when interpreting the dose-response curves. What is more is that these models used the crude endpoint (i.e., lung cancer), and no mechanistic information, such as the nature of the observed effect and an elucidation of the relevant pathways, was available for these cohorts to strengthen this evaluation. For all these reasons, the overall results presented in this chapter should be interpreted with caution, and care must be taken to avoid overgeneralizing the risk estimates.

An obvious concern in the interpretation of the results is whether the study design can affect the risk estimates or the shape of the dose-response curve. In this vein, in the VITAL study, the hazard ratio for lung cancer associated with 10-year use of supplemental vitamin E was as low as 0.80 (95% *CI*: 0.62-1.04) for a vitamin E use of 42-215 mg/d, *p* trend = .03 (slatore et al., 2008). The much lower hazard ratio for this group may be a consequence of the dose selection, type of dose (dietary/supplemental; dietary α-tochopherol/supplemental RRR-α-tocopherol/ VES), and dose levels used in this study compared to the study conducted by Wright et al. (2004). Therefore, it is believed that both the shape of the dose-response relationship and the risk estimates are sensitive to the study design, e.g., applied forms of vitamin E, applied doses, groups sizes, reference groups, and the survival times considered (i.e., the times of follow-up: 10 years versus 14.4 years); however, further research and more information are needed before any definitive statements can be made.

An important finding in this analysis is that vitamin E effects tended to have lower relative risk values than adjusted hazard ratios (see the above-mentioned tables). A possible explanation may be that the biochemical responses were measured in Wright et al. (2004) study, whereas more complex responses of vitamin E were observed by Slatore et al. (2008). To put it differently, the dose-response relationships responsible for the biochemical responses in Wright et al. study tended to be linear compared to the dose-response relationships for the complex, slightly toxicological responses observed by Slatore and coworkers. This result should be considered in light of the conclusions reached by other researchers. For example, Miller et al. (2005) reported that high-dosage vitamin E supplements (i.e., $\geq$ 400 IU/d) may increase all-cause mortality and should be avoided (Miller et al., 2005), while van Leeuwen and Vermeire (2007) suggested that a toxicological response can induce lung cancer if an individual is exposed to relatively high levels of vitamin E for prolonged periods of time (van Leeuwen & Vermeire, 2007). Under these circumstances, vitamin E may be involved in increased oxidative stress within the lung tissue and/or in the deregulation of the apoptotic pathways, thereby inducing cancer formation by providing tumor cells with a survival mechanism compared to their normal counterparts. Nevertheless, this statement should be considered tentative because it is based on inadequate evidence.

Aside from the points raised above, careful and critical attention should be given to extrapolation of the results presented in this chapter. More specifically, a subsequent evaluation of the study conducted by Wright et al. (2004) implied that the dose-response curve for the specified response was consistent with linearity over the range of doses tested. However, this does not imply that the curve would be linear outside the range of doses specified in the study. Consequently, in order to avoid extrapolation and to reduce the limitations of this kind of studies, future studies should be designed to fit a nonlinear regression model.

Overall, the aforementioned differences in dose-response relationships suggest a lack of a unified dose-response relationship between vitamin E use and lung cancer risk for these two studies. And yet, the lack of a joint dose-response relationship between the two studies is, by itself, not a valid reason to discredit the findings of the studies under evaluation. It is believed that different dose-response relationships may be observed if and when vitamin E use produces different biological effects (van Leeuwen & Vermeire, 2007). Dose-response relationships for relatively simple responses, such as receptor activation, may be different from dose-response relationships for apoptosis of lung cancer cells or toxicological (carcinogenic) responses. As it was demonstrated in this chapter, these studies suggest diverse dose-dependent patterns, which in turn may reflect differences in the methodologies applied and the estimates calculated, as well as differences in the mechanisms of action considered by the researchers.

CHAPTER 3: MECHANISM-BASED VITAMIN E-LUNG CANCER MODELS

Abstract

This chapter elucidates a better understanding of the possible anti-carcinogenic mechanism(s) of action of vitamin E with regards to lung cancer risk by exploring a number of pathways identified and discussed by epidemiologists and researchers in their search for evidence on the mechanisms of action of vitamin E in relation to lung cancer risk. Research findings on the biological and cellular effects of vitamin E indicate that there is a certain pattern between doses and responses over various time intervals. Vitamin E may possess the ability to induce lung cancer cells to undergo apoptosis, and stimulating specific proteins is the first step in a series of biological, cellular, and tissue-level reactions that ultimately lead to apoptotic cell death. The chapter attempts further to suggest a hypothesis that apoptotic signaling in lung cancer cells can be generated by a potential interaction between vitamin E and certain structural components of cell membranes, such as ceramides, thereby offering an alternative to the hypothesis that vitamin E usually induces apoptosis through the activation of Fas or the JNK signaling pathway.

Mechanism-Based Dose-Response Models

As opposed to empirical dose-response models, comprehensive mechanism-based dose-response models can yield a better understanding of the principles and mechanisms behind complex biological phenomena (Foch et al., 2000). However, any scientific uncertainty or misinterpretations with respect to the mechanisms that the models express will, without doubt, lead to uncertainty in the predictions presented by the models.

Generally, the response-dependent biological effects of vitamin E are considered to depend on dose, exposure duration, tissue, frequency (i.e., the number of repeated exposures), stress level, overall health status, genetic susceptibility, and environmental factors (van Leeuwen & Vermeire, 2007). In this context, the results of the literature review carried out emphasized that receptor activation is a vital step towards the induction of apoptosis in lung cancer cells (e.g., Kline et al., 2001). Furthermore, it has been documented that vitamin E can trigger apoptosis in breast cancer cells, but instead of inducing growth inhibition via the SMAD signaling pathway, it restores transforming growth factor-β (TGF-β) signaling, resulting in activation of the JNK signaling pathway (see the TGF-β and the DAXX pathways in the next section).

However, as noted above, the dose-response relationships that result in apoptosis are most likely different from the curves obtained from receptor activation effects. In addition to that, although a mechanism of receptor activation for breast cancer cells has been presented to the scientific community, this mechanism may not be applicable in the case of lung cancer. Also, other mechanisms of action may be involved, including SMAD, and Rac1 (see *SMAD pathway* and *sphingomylin pathway* in the next section). For instance, via interactions with cell-specific factors, vitamin E may enable lung cancer cells to activate receptor proteins located in the cell surface membrane, thereby inducing cell cycle arrest and preventing cell replication. What is more, the latency period of human lung cancer is about 20-40 years (Klassen, 2008), making its relationship to vitamin E as a specific exposure difficult to establish.

It must be borne in mind that various models, ranging from simple to complex, have been developed to describe the mechanism of action of vitamin E in relation to (lung) cancer risk. Clearly, the biology governing the protective effects of vitamin E on the incidence of lung cancer varies greatly from one study to another. Still, one common point is that the first essential event in this mechanism is response-independent and related to the activation of inactive ligand proteins.

Mechanism-Based Vitamin E-Lung Cancer Models

General Overview

The potential mechanisms of lung cancer have been studied extensively, suggesting that oxidative damage to DNA is a major cause of mutations that lead to lung cancer (Klassen, 2008). In this respect, it is important to underline that small changes in DNA structure can markedly influence carcinogenic potency and that tumor cells are likely to pass their abnormalities on to their daughter cells (Bignold, 2004). This implies that a genomic alteration may trigger tumor formation and, in so doing, transforming protooncogenes to oncogenes, i.e., any changes in the expression of the so-called protooncogenes (normal genes found in all cells and involved in the control of growth and development) may convert them into the cancer-causing genes called oncogenes (Bignold, 2004; Solomon et al, 1996). Further, it has been suggested that genetic instability might occur during the early phase of carcinogenesis (Takayama et al., 2001; Bignold, 2004). Also, many mutations (in both dominant and recessive oncogenes) have to develop until the cancer becomes fully invasive (Klassen, 2008). Nonetheless, we must remember that not all carcinogens are mutagens, and mutagens may or may not be carcinogens (Bignold, 2004).

Accordingly, uncontrolled cellular proliferation is a hallmark of (lung) cancer given that cancer cells lack normal biological inhibition (Gold, 1999; Solomon et al., 1996). The growth and division of normal lung cells are tightly regulated by control mechanisms triggered by one or more external signal molecules called growth factors that bind to specific growth factor receptors associated with the cell surface, initiating a cascade of events inside the cell, prompting them to divide when necessary and preventing their growth and division when inappropriate (Solomon et al., 1996). Thus, normal lung cells reproduce only to replace neighboring cells that have died or been damaged. In contrast, lung cancer cells escape such normal growth regulatory mechanisms and become malignant (Solomon et al., 1996). In other words, understanding the molecular events involved in growth regulatory proteins in normal cells and its lack of function in tumor cells should determine the potential mechanism(s) by which vitamin E may influence lung cancer risk. Therefore, the key questions that arise here are:

- How this lack of growth control in tumor cells happens?
- What events favor lung cancer formation?
- What events favor apoptotic cancer cell death?
- Is vitamin E involved in any or some of these events?
- And if it does, what are the pathways that mediate vitamin E action?

The molecular mechanism(s) by which vitamin E may exert an anti-carcinogenic effect are uncertain, but suggestions include:

- Inhibition of the oxidative modification of low density lipoprotein (Vitols et al., 1992; Williams et al., 1997; Niki et al., 1993);
- Vitamin E seems to have anti-mutagenic or anti-cancer activities. Dietary vitamin E offers strong protection against both spontaneously arising and nitric oxide-induced mutations by two distinct protective mechanisms, namely (i) scavenging of a nitric oxide-related genotoxic species and (ii) altering the infiltration of neutrophils into tumors (Sandhu et al., 2000); and

- Dietary intake of antioxidants appears to have observed effects on antioxidative enzyme activities (Hilbert & Mohsenin, 1996).

Most importantly, and as it will be discussed in the next subsections, vitamin E possesses numerous properties that are independent of its chain-breaking antioxidant ability, including an effect on protein kinase C activity, which is involved in cell proliferation, cell adhesion, enhancement of immune responses, free radical production, and gene expression (Ricciarelli et al., 2001; Wright et al., 2004). Additionally, in recent years, several studies have found that vitamin E can induce apoptosis in a large number of cancer cells; however, the exact pathways involved are yet to be elucidated (Comitato et al., 2009).

In order to understand the effects of vitamin E on lung cancer risk, it is necessary to understand what happens when adequate or high levels of vitamin E are taken on a regular basis. A case-control study conducted by Gromadzinska and colleagues (2003) indicated an increased concentration of vitamin E in the erythrocytes of lung cancer patients, which was suggested to indicate an intracellular accumulation of this compound (Gromadzinska et al., 2003). It is most likely that this process plays a protective role against free radical-induced damage (i.e., long-term oxidative stress). It follows that the fewer the free radicals, the less is the chance of developing lung cancer.

A significant study in this direction has been conducted by Hilbert and Mohsenin (1996), in which they showed that vitamin E concentration was markedly higher in smokers' lung lavage cells (403.3±81.0 in smokers versus 16.6±5.3 ng/10^6 cells in nonsmokers), and that bronchoalveolar lavage cell vitamin E increased from 403.3±81.0 to 477.4±97.7 ng/10^6 cells ($p < .05$) after starting the vitamin E supplements (Hilbert & Mohsenin, 1996). The authors suggested that exposure to oxidants and low concentration of vitamins in body fluids (BAL) is responsible for its intracellular accumulation (Hilbert & Mohsenin, 1996).

In light of these results, it seems reasonable to suggest that, taking account of other known risk factors (e.g., smoking and plasma levels of other anti-oxidative vitamins), low vitamin E intake may be regarded as a factor that increases lung cancer risk.

Vitamin E-Induced Tumor Cell Apoptosis

The ability of vitamin E in inducing lung cancer apoptosis is meant to be related to protein kinase C activity. This protein is a family of enzymes that play key regulatory roles in a multitude of cellular processes, ranging from control of simple cell autonomous activities (e.g., proliferation) to higher functions (e.g., memory formation) (Mellor & Parker, 1998; Capra et al., 2006). At least 125 of the over 500 human protein kinases are the Serine-Threonine Kinases (STKs) family that is believed to be involved in human cancers, and its main types include (i) receptor protein STKs (i.e., those acting directly as receptors); and (ii) intracellular signaling peptides and proteins (Capra et al., 2006). Research has found that alteration in the expression of STKs is a relatively frequent event in human tumors, and three specific patterns of alterations have been identified, namely (i) an overexpression in the absence of expression in the normal tissues (10 kinases), (ii) an overexpression in the presence of expression by normal tissues (8 kinases), and (iii) an underexpression (3 kinases) (Capra et al., 2006).

It must be noted here that apoptosis plays a central role in development, homeostasis (i.e., the body's ability to maintain an inner balance or a state of stability despite changing conditions in the environment), tumor surveillance, and the function of the immune system (Wajant, 2002). Two principal pathways, intrinsic and extrinsic pathways, initiate apoptosis. While the intrinsic pathway emerges from mitochondria and involves cytochrome *c* and SMAC/Diablo (see the next subsection), the extrinsic pathway is activated by the ligation of death receptors on the surface of cells, and one such receptor is Fas (Wajant, 2002).

Fas Signaling Pathway

Fas (Apo-1/CD95) is a cell-surface receptor involved in cell death signaling through binding of Fas ligand to Fas receptor. The Fas gene, which is comprised of 9 exons and 8 introns, is located on chromosome 10 (i.e., 10q24.1), and mutations of this gene might be involved in proliferative diseases as it prolongs the programmed death of certain cells (Takayama et al., 2001). This pathway is the most complete mechanism of action presented for vitamin E so far. The proposed pathway is illustrated in Figure 1 and can be described as follows:

Following Fas-FasL ligation, a complex of proteins associates with activated Fas results in the formation of Death-Inducing Signaling Complex (DISC) (Bobé, 2002). First of all, Fas-Associated protein with Death Domain (FADD) binds via its own death domain (DD) to the DD in Fas, while it binds via its own death-effector domain (DED) to the DED in procaspase-8 (also called the zymogen form of caspase-8 because it is the inactive precursor of caspase-8 and requires some change to become active), which in turn is activated, and the active enzyme caspase-8 (Cysteine Aspartate Specific ProteASE 8) is released from the DISC into the cytoplasm in the form of a heterotetramer of two small subunits (p10) and two large subunits (p20) (Bobé, 2002).

Fas-mediated apoptosis in type I cells (e.g., lymphoid cells) is initiated through the formation of large amounts of active caspase-8, followed by direct cleavage of procaspase-3, resulting in activated caspase-3 that has both the ability to (i) activate other caspases, such as procaspase-6 and -7, that subsequently degrade cellular targets that lead to cell death; and to (ii) cleave a variety of substrates, including DNA repair enzymes, cellular and nuclear structural proteins, and many other cellular constituents, such as Caspase-Activated Deoxyribonuclease (CAD), and Inhibitor Caspase-Activated Deoxyribonuclease (ICAD) (Bobé, 2002; CRI, n.d.).

Conversely, in type II cells, small amounts of active caspase-8 are formed, some of which cuts the Bcl-2 family member Bid, and the truncated Bid induces insertion of BAX into mitochondrial membrane in order to release pro-apoptotic molecules, including cytochrome c and SMAC/Diablo (Bobé, 2002; CRI, n.d.). While cytochrome c is a protein that helps mitochondria generate ATP (Weaver & Hedrick, 1997), SMAC/Diablo is a protein released from mitochondria into the cytosol (i.e., the intracellular fluid) in response to apoptotic stimuli (Sun et al., 2008). The latter inhibits the activity of a potent suppressor of apoptotic cell death called X-linked inhibitor of apoptosis protein (XIAP); hence, cell death is promoted because XIAP is suppressed (Bobé, 2002; CRI, n.d.; Sun et al., 2008). In other words, apoptosis is regulated by the interplay between pro- and anti-apoptotic members of the Bcl-2 family (Aurelian, 2005). Pro-apoptotic members include Bax, Bad, Bid, Bim and Bik, and contain an α-helical BH3 DD that binds to anti-apoptotic family members Bcl-2 and Bcl-$_{XL}$, forming heterodimers that block their survival activity; hence, the relative abundance of pro- and anti-apoptotic Bcl-2 family members determines the overall susceptibility of lung cells to programmed death (Aurelian, 2005). Taken together, these reports provide evidence that blocking activation of mitochondria by Bcl-2 or Bcl-x_L inhibits apoptosis only in type II cells.

The last steps in this pathway involve the activation of caspase-9 by cytochrome c, and together with apoptosis protease-activating factor 1 (Apaf-1) apoptosome is formed, and this large protein is capable of activating further downstream procaspase-3 (Bobé, 2002; CRI, n.d.).

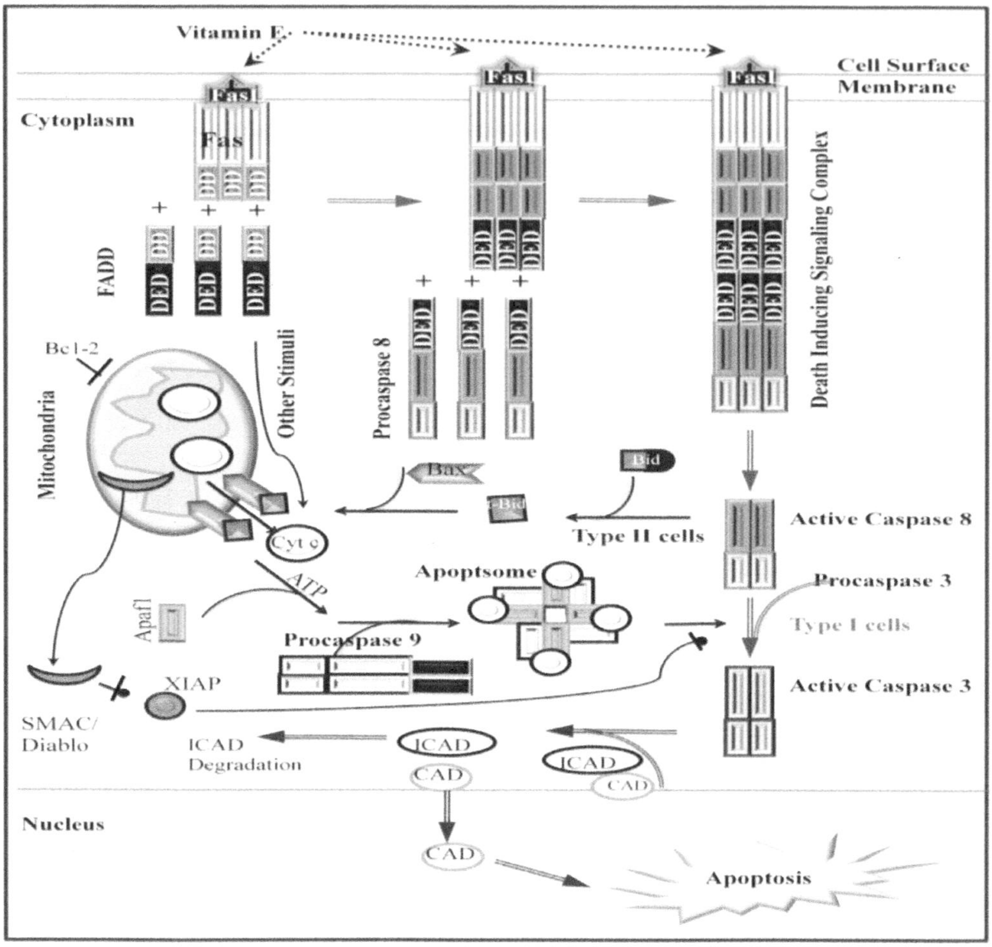

Figure 1. Schematic representation of the Fas-FADD signaling pathway. Extracellular signals, such as the presence of vitamin E, can trigger apoptosis via two different pathways. Activation of Fas by Fas ligand (Fas L) induces recruitment of FADD to the receptor complex via homologous death domain (DD) interactions. This complex binds via death effector domain (DED) to procaspase-8, inducing proteolytic activation to p10 and p20 subunits and forming the death-inducing signaling complex (DISC). In type II cells, the little DISC formed leads to the activation of mitochondria by cleaving the Bid protein. The

resulting truncated Bid (t-Bid) inactivates Bcl-2, causing the release of cytochrome c and SMAC/Diablo from the mitochondria and inactivating inhibitors of apoptosis. Cytochrome c clusters with Apaf-1 and procaspase-9 in the presence of ATP to activate caspase-9. In contrast, in type I cells, CD95 triggering leads to strong caspase-8 activation by large amounts of DISC formation, and active caspase-8 bypasses mitochondria directly, leading to the activation of caspase-3, the breakdown of caspase-activated deoxyribonuclease (CAD) inhibitor (ICAD), the degradation of ICAD, the translocation of CAD to the nucleus, and subsequently to apoptosis. Light grey box, death domain; black box, death effector domain.

Transforming Growth Factor-β Pathways

Transforming growth factor-betas (TGF-βs) are one of few classes of endogenous inhibitors of cell growth. These polypeptide proteins are secreted as inactive (latent) precursors in large protein complexes and exert extensive control over all aspects of development, and components of this pathway are frequently mutated in cancers and in several hereditary disorders (Sterner-Kock et al., 2002; Wrana, 2000; Gold, 1999). These multifunctional complexes include the latency-associated propeptide (LAP) and a latent transforming growth factor-β binding protein (LTBP) (Sterner-Kock et al., 2002). So far, four isoforms of LTBPs (LTBP-1-LTBP-4) have been cloned, and they are believed to have a dual role as structural components of connective tissue microfibrils and as local regulators of TGF-β tissue deposition and signaling (Sterner-Kock et al., 2002).

Contrary to the first notion that these growth factor proteins may be down-regulated in (lung) cancer cells to promote their growth, it has been otherwise found that there is a marked increase in the expression of TGF-β mRNA and protein in human cancers (in vivo), including those of the lung, prostate, and breast (Gold, 1999). Additionally, in many types of cancers, high expression correlates with more advanced stages of malignancy and decreased survival, i.e., the increased expression of TGF-βs is often accompanied by a loss in the growth inhibitory response to TGF-βs (Gold, 1999). Once malignant cells lose their growth inhibitory response to TGF-βs and produce massive amounts of these proteins, this increased expression provides a selective advantage for tumor cell survival, mainly because TGF-βs have also angiogenic and immunosuppressive effects, including inhibition of tumoricidal natural and lymphocyte-activated killer cells (Gold, 1999). The significant aspect of this discussion is that research has shown that a disruption in the human *LTBP-4* gene results in severe pulmonary emphysema, leading to highly tissue-specific abnormalities, primarily due to profound defects in the elastic fiber structure and a reduced deposition of TGF-β in the extracellular space, and eventually these epithelial cells with reduced levels of phosphorylated SMAD2 proteins (i.e., amino acid proteins involved in cell signaling) overexpress the cell cycle stimulator c-myc and undergo uncontrolled proliferation (Sterner-Kock et al., 2002). In light of these observations, there is a need to underline that epithelial cells are one of the 4 main bodily tissues; they line the insides of the lungs, and simple squamous epithelium, which are composed of flat cells and are arranged as single layer, are found lining the air sacs of lungs and the alveolar epithelium *(i.e.,* the respiratory epithelial barrier) in the lungs (Solomon et al., 1997). In general terms, TGF-β can induce apoptosis in two different pathways: SMAD and DAXX pathways.

SMAD pathway. SMADs are a small family of transcription regulators that are involved in cell signaling, in particular in the transforming growth factor-β signaling cascade (Hariharan & Pillai, 2008; Massagué et al., 2005). Essentially, apart from TGF-β, the TGF-β superfamily also includes factors, such as the activins (i.e., dimmers composed of two identical or very similar TGF-β subunits that are linked to one another by a single disulfide bond) and the bone morphogenetic proteins; these factors signal through heteromeric complexes of type II and type I STK receptors, which activate the downstream SMAD signal transduction pathway (see Figure 2) (Wrana, 2000; Ying, 1987).

Researchers have identified three classes of SMADs (Wrana, 2000; Ishisaki et al., 1999; Wharton & Derynck, 2009; Hariharan & Pillai, 2008):

1) Receptor-regulated SMADs (R-SMADs), such as SMAD1-SMAD3 and SMAD5;
2) Common-mediator SMADs (co-SMADs), such as SMAD4, which interacts with R-SMADs to affect TGF-β signaling; and

3) Antagonistic or inhibitory SMADs (I-SMADs), such as SMAD6 and SMAD7, both of which inhibit signaling downstream of TGF-β type I receptors, thereby preventing ligand-induced activation of signaling mediated by TGF-β superfamily of ligands. Compared to SMAD6, SMAD7 has a more flexible overall folding, characterized by amino acid residues that are located on highly flexible and functionally important regions (Hariharan & Pillai, 2008).

TGF-βs carry out tumor suppressor activity in epithelial and lymphoid cells, which may be in part mediated by repressing telomerase activity that is required for most cancers (Li et al., 2006). Specifically, SMAD3 (also known as mothers against decapentaplegic homolog 3) is involved in inducing apoptosis through modulating signals of activin and TGF-βs; it binds to SMAD4 and after entering the nucleus, it forms complexes with other proteins and acts as a transcription factor (Li & Liu, 2008). Figure 2 shows that the SMADs, by forming a trimer of two R-SMADs and a co-SMAD (SMAD4), act as transcription factors with varying abilities, including the regulation of the expression of certain genes (Massagué et al., 2005; Wrana, 2000).

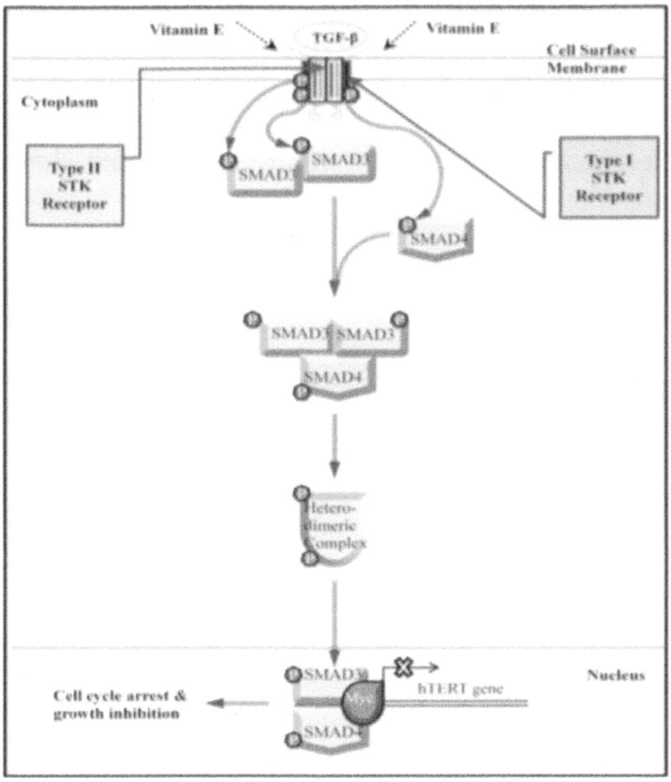

Figure 2. Schematic representation of the TGF-β signaling pathway or the SMAD signaling pathway. It is hypothesized that vitamin E treatment activates TGF-β dimers to bind to a type II receptor which recruits and phosphorylates a type I receptor, which in turn recruits and phosphorylates SMADs, forming heterodimeric complexes. These SMAD complexes enter the nucleus where they interact with c-myc, repress the *c-myc* gene, bind to *hTERT* gene promoter, and inhibit *hTERT* gene transcription activity, resulting in cell cycle arrest and growth inhibition.

More specifically, complexes of type II and type I STK receptors activate the SMAD pathway by interacting and phosphorylating specific R-SMADs in the cytoplasm, i.e., TGF-β dimers bind to a type II receptor which recruits and phosphorylates a type I receptor, which in turn recruits and phosphorylates an R-SMAD (Wrana, 2000). The latter will then bind to SMAD4, a co-SMAD, and form a heterodimeric complex, which enters the cell nucleus where the SMADs activate apoptosis by playing a key role as transcription factors for several genes, such as the ones that activate the MAPK pathway (Wrana, 2000; Li & Liu, 2008). For instance, they interact with c-myc and repress the *c-myc* gene; they also bind to human telomerase reverse transcriptase (hTERT) gene promoter directly and inhibit *hTERT* gene transcription activity (Li & Liu, 2008). In other words, TGF-β prevents continuous cell proliferation by switching off telomerase activity through SMAD3's repression of these two genes (Li & Liu, 2008).

DAXX pathway. In addition to SMAD pathway, TGF-β can also trigger apoptosis via the DAXX pathway.

DAXX protein. The first component of this pathway is related to the Death Associated protein 6 (DAXX adapter protein), which is encoded by the *DAXX* gene and resides in multiple locations in the nucleus and in the cytoplasm (NCBI, 2011; Yang et al., 1997). In the nucleus, DAXX functions as a potent transcription repressor that binds to sumoylated transcription factors, while in the cytoplasm, it interacts with a wide range of proteins, including binding to the Fas cell surface receptor – a signaling process that induces apoptosis (NCBI, 2011;

Yang et al., 1997). As seen in Figure 3, overexpression of DAXX enhances Fas-mediated programmed cell death and activates both MAPK cascades and the c-Jun N-terminal Kinase (JNK) pathway (Yang et al., 1997). Whereas a C-terminal portion of DAXX interacts with the Fas death receptor, a different region activates both JNK and apoptosis (Yang et al., 1997). The DAXX apoptotic pathway is sensitive to both Bcl-2 and dominant-negative JNK pathway components and acts cooperatively with the Fas-Associated protein with Death Domain (FADD) pathway. Hence, DAXX and FADD define two distinct apoptotic pathways downstream of Fas (Yang et al., 1997).

MAPK cascades. The second component of the DAXX pathway is related to MAPK cascades. Types of intracellular signaling STKs include Mitogen-Activated Protein Kinases (MAPKs), which can be defined as STKs that are responding to extracellular stimuli (e.g., mitogens) (Pearson et al., 2001). Typical MAPK cascades (i.e., stimulus-GTPase-MAPK4-MAPK3-MAPK2-MAPK) plays a crucial role in many aspects of immune mediated inflammatory responses and regulate various cellular activities, such as gene expression, mitosis (growth), differentiation, and cell survival/apoptosis (see the DAXX pathway below) (Pearson et al., 2001; Kline et al., 2001).

JNK pathway. The third component of the DAXX pathway is related to the JNK pathway. It is of importance to mention here that DAXX does not activate the JNK pathway by itself, but rather the upstream JNK kinase kinase ASK1 (Apoptosis Signal-regulating Kinase 1), also known as Mitogen-Activated

Protein Kinase Kinase Kinase 5 (MAP3K5) (Bobé, 2002). Or, in other terms, JNK activates HIPK2, a conserved serine-threonine nuclear kinase, which stands for the translocation of nuclear DAXX to the cytoplasm, where it also can activate ASK1.

The HIPK2/p53 pathway. The last component of the DAXX pathway is related to HIPK2 and *p53* gene. DAXX can interact and suppress several transcription factors, such as the p53 oncosuppressor protein. This is a very important tumor suppressor gene because at least 40% of sporadic (nonfamilial) cancers involve a defective *p53* gene (Weaver & Hedrick, 1997). Under normal circumstances, p53 is negatively regulated through a partnership with MDM2, an ubiquitin regulatory protein that binds to p53 and labels it for destruction (Di Stefano et al., 2004).

In contrast, following stress and/or DNA damage, p53 undergoes post-translational modifications that allow this protein to escape MDM2 control, accumulate rapidly, become active, and binds to HIPK2, which phosphorylates p53 (Di Stefano et al., 2004), inducing p53 transcriptional activity and its two different functions. Firstly, after sensing DNA damage, p53 blocks DNA replication and cell division until the damage is repaired, which prevents the creation of a permanent mutation (Weaver & Hedrick, 1997). Secondly, if this blockade of cell division fails, p53 induces apoptosis, i.e., it causes the cell with the damaged DNA to "commit suicide," thereby suppressing tumorigenesis (Weaver & Hedrick, 1997). Thus, the p53 pathway is a highly regulated process that determines cell fate.

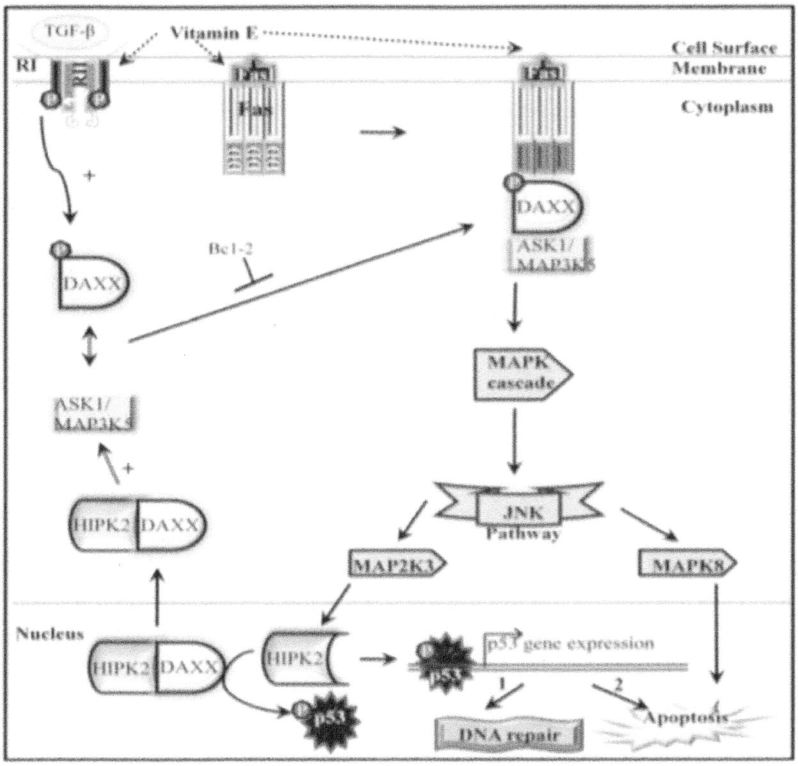

Figure 3. Schematic representation of DAXX, JNK, and p53 pathways. Activation of the MAPK cascades generally results in apoptosis through a multi-step process. JNK pathway responds to extraneous signals, including vitamin E presence. These signals activate HIPK2, which translocates nuclear DAXX to the cytoplasm, where DAXX activates ASK1 (also known as MAP3K5), binds to Fas cell surface receptor, thereby enhancing Fas-mediated programmed cell death and activating JNK pathway. Bcl-2 has the ability to inhibit DAXX pathway. In the p53 pathway, upon DNA damage or signs of cancer cells, transcription factor p53 binds to HIPK2, which phosphorylates p53, inducing p53 transcriptional activity

and its dual functions, (1) the induction of a cell cycle arrest to allow DNA repair and survival of the cell or (2) apoptosis to discard the damaged cell.

Sphingolipid Pathway: Effects Of γ-Tocopherol On Prostate Cancer Cells

On a related front, combinations of some vitamin E isomers, such as gamma-tocopherol (γ-T) and δ-tocopherol, have been found capable of inducing cell death in human prostate cancer cells by interrupting the de novo sphingolipid pathway, i.e., by the induction of cytochrome c release, activation of caspase-9 and caspase-3, cleavage of poly-ADP-ribose polymerase (PARP), and involvement of caspase-independent pathways (Jiang et al., 2004). Researchers like Jiang team (2004) have demonstrated that vitamin E (γ-T) treatment can lead to pronounced dihydroceramide and dihydrosphingosine accumulation, which precede morphological and biochemical manifestations of apoptosis (Jiang et al., 2004). They found that only myriocin and fumonisin B1, the specific inhibitors of key enzymes (serine palmitoyltransferase and dihydroceramide synthase, respectively) in de novo synthesis of sphingolipids, can significantly protect these cells from γ-T-induced DNA fragmentation, cytochrome c release, PARP cleavage, and the formation of active caspase-3 (Jiang et al., 2004).

This means that certain vitamin E isomers or mixed forms of vitamin E may be valuable as anti-cancer agents. Also, it is believed that γ-tocopherol (the predominant form of vitamin E in diets), but not α-tocopherol (the major vitamin E form in tissues and supplements), can inhibit proliferation of lung cancer cells

(A549) (Jiang et al., 2004). In addition, because research has highlighted that vitamin E has the ability to induce the JNK pathway through the activation of certain receptor proteins and since ceramides have the ability to induce the JNK pathway, it can be hypothesized that vitamin E intake (or intake of mixed forms of vitamin E) may induce apoptosis by inducing the generation of ceramides. This means that the sphingomyelin signal transduction pathway is considered of relevant importance for the purpose of this chapter; it will therefore be discussed in more details.

Sphingomyelin Signal Transduction Pathway

Sphingomyelin, which usually consists of phosphorylcholine and ceramide, is one of the four common phospholipids found in the plasma membrane of cells (Zhang et al., 1997). Previous research has shown that the sphingomyelin signal transduction pathway mediates apoptosis for Tumor Necrosis Factor α (TNF-α) in several nonhematopoietic cells (Haimovitz-Friedman, 1994; Zhang et al., 1997). In this pathway (see Figure 4), TNF-receptor interaction initiates sphingomyelin hydrolysis to ceramide by the enzyme sphingomyelinase (Haimovitz- Friedman, 1994). As a second messenger, ceramide stimulates a ceramide-activated STK protein (Haimovitz-Friedman, 1994).

Since sphingomyelin is found in cell membranes, the cellular membrane would be the target of extracellular signals that may positively or negatively regulate apoptosis induction. Previous investigations also provide evidence that TNF or UV light activate sphingomyelinase that leads to the generation of ceramide, resulting in the activation of a serine protease termed AP24 and DNA fragmentation in sensitive cells (Wright et al., 1996). While protein kinase C activation can block both radiation-induced sphingomyelin hydrolysis and apoptosis, apoptosis can be restored by ceramide analogues (Haimovitz-Friedman, 1994). Ceramides can be generated through three major pathways, namely the aforementioned sphingomyelinase pathway, the de novo pathway, and the Salvage pathway (Chalfant & Poeta, 2010). While ceramides are created from less complex molecules in the de novo pathway, they are generated through breaking down complex sphingolipids in the Salvage pathway (Chalfant & Poeta, 2010).

Rac1 Pathway

Another important pathway, which is also related to ceramide generation, is the Rac1pathway (see Figure 4 below). Rac1 is a member of the family of human Rho GTPases, which are critical elements in signal transduction pathways controlling cell proliferation and cell death (Embade et al., 2000).

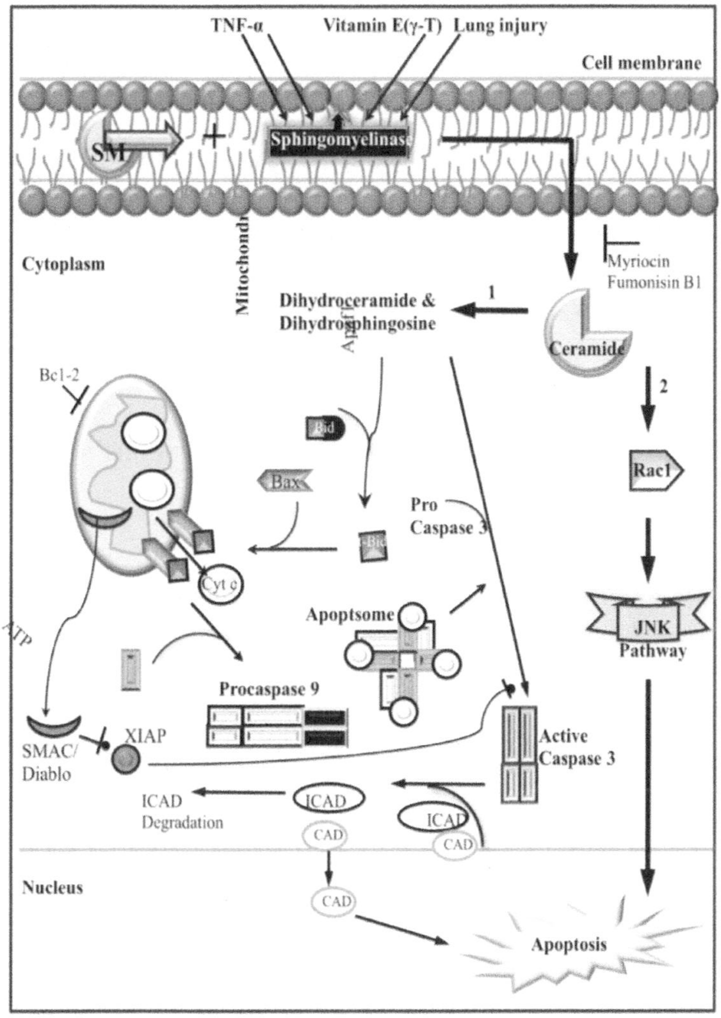

Figure 4. Schematic representation of sphingomyelin and Rac-1 pathways showing the hydrolysis of sphingomyelin (SM) through activation of sphingomyleniase. Signals, such as vitamin E treatment (γ-T) and several causes of lung injury, including Tumor Necrosis Factor α (TNF-α), can generate ceramide via SM cleavage. In this pathway, ceramide will either lead to

pronounced dihydroceramide and dihydrosphingosine accumulation, which induces apoptosis through Bax and Bak. Cytochrome c will be released from mitochondria and the caspase-dependent pathways will be activated. Specific inhibitors, such as myriocin and fumonisin B1, can inhibit these activities at several levels. Alternatively, ceramide can up-regulate the GTP-binding protein Rac-1, which induces the JNK pathway, ultimately leading to apoptosis.

Rac1-induced apoptosis is linked to the simultaneous increase in ceramide production and synthesis of FasL, and in most cases, the increased generation of FasL may be mediated by transcriptional regulation involving both c-Jun amino terminal kinase as well as nuclear factor-kappa B-dependent signals (Embade et al., 2000). Any of these two signals, ceramides or FasL, can be sufficient to induce apoptosis in the Rac1-expressing cells (Embade et al., 2000).

Discussion

In reviewing the previous sections, it is important to recognize that vitamin E mechanisms of action may involve the following genes: *hTERT* and *c-myc*; and the following proteins: FasL, TGF-β ligand, SMADs, DAXX, FADD, cytochrome c, HIPK2, p53, and several procaspases. It can be hypothesized that vitamin E intake or consumption of various isomers of vitamin E may positively or negatively regulate apoptosis induction through the possible induction or inhibition of the sphingomyelin signal transduction pathway and/or Rac1 pathway.It has been pointed out that vitamin E may trigger TGF-β signaling and Fas signaling pathways, leading to cell cycle arrest. Both TGF-β signaling and Fas signaling play important roles in tumorigenesis and carcinogenesis. During malignant progression, tumor cells are prone to resist the growth-inhibitory effects of TGF-β (i.e., the TGF-β's anti-proliferative effects), which may lead to uncontrolled proliferation. Although the mechanisms involved in this process are yet to be clearly defined, an up-regulation of both ligand and receptors is often observed. There are indications that vitamin E succinate treatment of these cells activates the ligand and up-regulates membrane TGF-β receptor II levels (Kline et al., 2001). And yet, instead of inducing growth inhibition via the SMAD signaling pathway, vitamin E's restoration of TGF-β signaling is thought to induce apoptosis through activating the JNK signaling pathway (Kline et al., 2001).With that being said, it is vital to note that recent research has implicated sphingomyelin hydrolysis and generation of ceramides as important regulatory pathways in apoptosis. As implied earlier, ceramides are found within the cell membrane of lung cells, i.e., they are one of the component lipids that make up sphingomyelin, which is one of the major lipids in the lipid bilayer. They can act as signaling molecules and their functions vary from regulating the proliferation and apoptosis (Chalfant & Poeta, 2010). The interaction between vitamin E and certain proteins may initiate the generation of ceramides, and the elevation of ceramide with exogenous ceramide analogues is reported to be sufficient to induce apoptosis (Haimovitz-Friedman et al., 1994). In addition to that, it is believed that Rac1 is capable of inducing apoptosis through a complex mechanism that involves the generation of ceramides and the de novo synthesis of FasL, and apoptosis mediated by Rac1 can result from a signaling mechanism that involves biochemical and transcriptional events controlled by Rac1 (Embade et al., 2000).

CHAPTER 4: CONCLUSION AND IMPLICATIONS

Even in this age of scientific progress, there are many biological phenomena that do not have a satisfactory scientific explanation. It is not yet possible to provide accurate estimates about the effects of micronutrient intake, especially vitamin E intake, on lung cancer risk; nevertheless, extensive research has revealed the need to explore all possible ways in which diet, supplement use, and other lifestyle and environmental factors may play a role in the development of lung cancer.

In terms of the effects of vitamin E on lung cancer risk, explanations have been offered as to whether vitamin E intake is associated with the risk of developing lung cancer, and suggestions has been given to identify the biological pathways connecting vitamin E intake to lung cancer risk. Researchers have, however, reached no definitive conclusions. For instance, Slatore et al. (2008) found that the long-term use of supplemental vitamin E was associated with a small increased risk of developing lung cancer, whereas Wright et al. (2004)

concluded that a balanced diet rich in a variety of antioxidant nutrients may be beneficial in reducing lung cancer risk. However, there are still areas that should be further examined, especially because the observed benefits have been modest and the increased risk observed has been small. With that in mind and given the worldwide prevalence of the disease, it seems prudent to analyze the dose-response relationship of vitamin E intake and lung cancer risk.

In this vein, to assess the dose-response relationship of dietary and supplemental intakes of vitamin E with regards to lung cancer risk, two main questions were raised in this book: What is the critical dose at which no beneficial effects of vitamin E are observed? And what is the shape of the dose-response curve for lung cancer risk at various doses of vitamin E? Despite their importance, these questions were difficult to address because of (i) the multiplicity of the effects that vitamin E exerts on human body; (ii) the complexity of the mechanisms involved; and (iii) the long latency of lung cancer. In other words, barriers to allowing a better understanding of the dose-response relationship between vitamin E intake and lung cancer risk include the multifactorial nature of lung cancer etiology, injury and repair mechanisms; the various isomers of vitamin E and their different biological activities and bioavailability; factors affecting tissue and serum vitamin E concentrations; factors influencing the absorption and distribution of dietary versus supplemental vitamin E intake; controversies about the shape of the dose-response curves; the strength of association between vitamin E intake and lung cancer risk; and the biological and molecular mechanisms involved.

Despite these barriers, it is important to point out that the current approach to lung cancer prevention is likely to be replaced in the future by a more effective and "proactive" approach, guided by an established set of policies and procedures that are grounded in scientific evidence, part of which may involve dose-response assessments, and biological processes that may occur in individuals at risk of lung cancer.

In the dose-response assessment conducted in this book, the best available statistical procedures were compared to identify the best tools that could provide appropriate risk estimates and ensure that the aforementioned questions would be properly answered. The book provides an extensive summary of dose-response models of vitamin E in lung cancer patients. The analyses and discussions presented here offer considerable, and at times novel, insights into the mechanisms of action of vitamin E. Several parts of the book highlight the depth and breadth of available data and model types proposed in research, identify the gaps in qualitative and quantitative research, and recognize the research needed to fill these gaps and to overcome some of the weaknesses and limitations of earlier studies. In view of the results presented in previous chapters, the following conclusions are drawn:

1) Dose-response models are the first steps towards a predictive theory of the possible protective effects of vitamin E intake on lung cancer risk.
2) Past research has reported that adequate intakes of dietary and

supplemental vitamin E is beneficial and may reduce the risk of developing lung cancer. More specifically, the estimated beneficial doses of supplemental vitamin E among men and women and those of dietary vitamin E among male smokers were 42-215 mg per day and 15-26.74 mg per day, respectively. However, when vitamin E intake reached a certain level (dose), it became toxic and was believed to slightly increase the risk of developing lung cancer (Wright et al., 2004; Slatore et al., 2008). The estimated critical doses of supplemental vitamin E among men and women and those of dietary vitamin E among male smokers were greater than 215 mg per day and 30.06 mg per day, respectively.

3) Biological responses to vitamin E are more likely to be linear within the safe or beneficial dose range, whereas the more complex responses, including toxicological responses are more likely to assume a nonlinear shape.
4) Exposure duration may affect not only the response observed, but also the pathways through which vitamin E exerts its possible effect. Responses, such as preventing lung cancer, may require prolonged activation of specific pathways before a potential benefit is detected.
5) The activation of the TGF-β and/or Fas R by the presence of vitamin E appears to initiate a cascade of events, resulting in an interaction between receptors and proteins involved in various biological and cellular responses, such as cell cycle regulation, growth inhibition, and apoptosis.

Many of these biochemical changes, predominantly the formation of death-inducing signaling complexes and the activation of JNK pathway, may mediate the protective effects of vitamin E.

6) Last but not least, a range of other biochemical changes, including the activation of sphingomyelin signal transduction pathway and Rac1 pathway, can be hypothesized as novel signaling pathways involved in the mechanism of action of vitamin E, but are yet to be fully examined.

REFERENCES

Allison, P. D. *(2003). Survival analysis using SAS.* Cary, NC: SAS Institute Inc.

Aurelian, L. (2005). Cross talk of signaling and apoptotic cascades in the CNS: Target for virus modulation. *Front Biosci., 10,* 2776-87.

Bewick, V., Cheek, L., & Ball, J. (2004). Statistics review 12: Survival analysis. *Critical Care, 8,* 389-394.

Bignold, L. P. (2004). Carcinogen-induced impairment of enzymes for replicative fidelity of DNA and the initiation of tumours. *Carcinogenesis 25(3),* 299-307.

Bobé, P. (2002). *The Fas - Fas Ligand apoptotic pathway.* Atlas Genet Cytogenet Oncol Haematol. Retrieved on March 10, 2011 at: http://atlasgeneticsoncology.org/Deep/Fas-FasLigandID20040.html

Bonamin, L. V. (2008). *Signals and images: Contributions and contradictions about high dilution research*. Brazil: Springer Science + Business Media B. V.

Cancer Research Institute (CRI) (n.d.). *Apoptosis Analysis*. Retrieved on March 10, 2011 at: http://qcri.queensu.ca/Apoptosis_Analysis_-112315.html

Capra, M., Nuciforo, P. G., Confalonieri, S., Quarto, M., Bianchi, M., Nebuloni, M.,… Di Fiore, P. P. (2006). Frequent alterations in the expression of serine/threonine kinases in human cancers. *Cancer Res., 66(16),* 8147-54.

Chalfant, C., & Poeta, M. D. (Eds.) (2010). *Sphingolipids as signaling and regulatory molecules*. USA: Landes Bioscience and Springer Science + Business Media, LLC.

Comitato, R., Nesaretnam, K., Leoni, G., Ambra, R., Canali, R., Bolli, A.,… Virgili F. (2009). A novel mechanism of natural vitamin E tocotrienol activity: Involvement of ER{beta} signal transduction. *Am. J. Physiol. Endocrinol. Metab., 297(2),* E427-E437.

Cox, D. R. *(1972).* Regression models and life tables (with Discussion). *Journal of the Royal Statistical Society Series B 34 (2),* 187-220.

Di Stefano, V., Blandino, G., Sacchi, A., Soddu, S., & D'Orazi, G. (2004). HIPK2 neutralizes MDM2 inhibition rescuing p53 transcriptional activity and apoptotic function. *Oncogene., 23(30),* 5185-5192.

Dietary Reference Intakes (DRIs) (2004). *Recommended intakes for individuals.* USA: Institute of Medicine of the U.S. National Academy of Sciences. Retrieved August 11, 2010, from http://www.iom.edu/Global/News%20Announcements/~/media/Files/Activity%20Files/Nutrition/DRIs/DRISummaryListing2.ashx

Embade, N., Valerón, P. F., Aznar, S., López-Collazo, E., & Lacal, J. C. (2000). Apoptosis induced by Rac GTPase correlates with induction of FasL and ceramides production. *Mol Biol Cell., 11(12),* 4347-4358.

Foch, B. J., McManus, H. L., & Cunningham, R. A. (2000). Mechanism-based modeling of long-term degradation. *Journal of Composites Technology & Research, 22 (3),* 146-152.

Gold, L. I. (1999). The role for transforming growth factor-beta (TGF-beta) in human cancer. *Crit Rev Oncog., 10(4),* 303-360.

Goutelle, S., Maurin, M., Rougier, F., Barbaut, X., Bourguignon, L., Ducher, M., & Maire P. (2008). The Hill equation: A review of its capabilities in pharmacological modelling. *Fundam Clin Pharmacol., 22(6),* 633-648.

Gromadzinska, J., Wasowicz, W., Rydzynski, K, & Szeszenia-Dabrowska, N. (2003). Oxidative-stress markers in blood of lung cancer patients occupationally exposed to carcinogens. *Biol Trace Elem Res., 91(3),* 203-215.

Haimovitz-Friedman, A., Kan, C. C., Ehleiter, D., Persaud, R. S., McLoughlin, M., Fuks, Z., & Kolesnick, R. N. (1994). Ionizing radiation acts on cellular membranes to generate ceramide and initiate apoptosis. *J. Exp. Med., 180 (2)*, 525-535.

Hariharan, R, & Pillai, M. R. (2008). Structure-function relationship of inhibitory Smads: Structural flexibility contributes to functional divergence. *Proteins, 71(4),* 1853-1862.

Hilbert, J., & Mohsenin, V. (1996). Adaptation of lung antioxidants to cigarette smoking in humans. *Chest, 110,* 16-20.

Hoel, D. G. (1980). Incorporation of background in dose-response models. *Federation Proceedings, 39,*73-75.

Husgafvel-Pursiainen, K., & Kannio, A. (1996). Cigarette smoking and p53 mutations in lung cancer and bladder cancer. Environ Health Perspect., *104(3),* 553-556.

Ishisaki, A., Yamato, K., Hashimoto, S., Nakao, A., Tamaki, K., Nonaka, K.,… Nishihara, T. (1999). Differential inhibition of Smad6 and Smad7 on bone morphogenetic protein- and activin-mediated growth arrest and apoptosis in B cells. *J Biol Chem., 274(19),* 13637-13642.

Jiang, Q., Wong, J., Fyrst, H., Saba, J. D., & Ames, B. N. *(2004).* Gamma-tocopherol or combinations of vitamin E forms induce cell death in human prostate cancer cells by interrupting sphingolipid synthesis. *Proc Natl Acad Sci USA, 101(51),* 17825-17830.

Key, T.J., Allen, N.E., Spencer, E.A., & Travis, R.C. (2002). The effect of diet on risk of cancer. *The Lancet, 360,* 861-868.

Klassen, C. D. (2008). *Casarett and Doull's toxicology: The basic science of poisons*. USA: Library of Congress Cataloging in Publication Data.

Li, H., & Liu, J. P. (2008). Mechanisms of action of TGF-beta in cancer: Evidence for Smad3 as a repressor of the hTERT gene. *Ann. N. Y. Acad. Sci., 1114,* 56-68.

Li, H., Xu, D., Toh, B. H., & Liu, J. P. (2006). TGF-beta and cancer: Is Smad3 a repressor of hTERT gene? *Cell Res., 16(2),* 169-173.

Mandema, J. W., Hermann, D., Wang, W., Sheiner, T., Milad, M., Bakker-Arkema, R., & Hartman, D. (2005). Model-based development of gemcabene, a new lipid-altering agent. *American Association of Pharmaceutical Scientists J., 7(3),* E513-E522.

Massagué, J., Seoane, J., & Wotton, D. (2005). Smad transcription factors. *Genes Dev., 19 (23),* 2783-2810.

MedCalc (2011). *Cox proportional-hazards regression*. Retrieved on March 15, 2011 at: http://www.medcalc.org/manual/cox_proportional_hazards.php

MedlinePlus (2013). *Gene study uncovers origins of many common cancers.* Retrieved on August 16, 2013 at: http://www.nlm.nih.gov/medlineplus/news/fullstory_139759.html

Mellor, H., & Parker, P. J. (1998). The extended protein kinase C superfamily. *Biochem. J.,* 332 (Pt 2), 281-292.

Miller, E. R. 3rd, Pastor-Barriuso, R., Dalal, D., Riemersma, R. A., Appel, L. J., & Guallar, E. (2005). Meta-analysis: High-dosage vitamin E supplementation may increase all-cause mortality. *Ann Intern Med., 142(1),* 37-46.

National Academy of Sciences (NAS) (1994). *Science and judgment in risk assessment.* USA, Washington D.C.: National Academy Press.

National Center for Biotechnology Information (NCBI) (2011). DAXX *death-domain associated protein [Homo sapiens].* Retrieved on February 7, 2011 at: http://www.ncbi.nlm.nih.gov/sites/entrez?Db=gene&Cmd=ShowDetailView&TermToSearch=1616

Niki, E., Noguchi, N., & Gotoh, N. (1993). Inhibition of oxidative modification of low density lipoprotein by antioxidants. *J Nutr Sci Vitaminol, 39 Suppl,* S1-8.

Pearson, G., Robinson, F., Beers Gibson, T., Xu, B. E., Karandikar, M., Berman,

K. & Cobb, M. H. (2001). Mitogen-activated protein (MAP) kinase pathways: Regulation and physiological functions. *Endocr. Rev., 22(2),* 153-183.

Roth, J, & Grunfield, C. (1985). *Mechanism of action of peptide hormones and catecholamines*. Philadelphia: W. B. Saunders.

Sandhu, J. K., Haqqani, A. S., & Birnboim, H. C. (2000). Effect of dietary vitamin E on spontaneous or nitric oxide donor-induced mutations in a mouse tumor model. *J Natl Cancer Inst., 92(17),*1429-1433.

Satia-About a, J., Patterson, R. E., King, I. B., Stratton, K. L., Shattuck, A. L., Kristal, A. R.,… White, E. (2003). Reliability and validity of self-report of vitamin and mineral supplement use in the vitamins and lifestyle study. *Am J Epidemiol, 157,* 944-954.

Slatore, C. G., Littman, A. J., Au, D. H, & White, E. (2008). Long-term use of supplemental multivitamins, vitamin C, vitamin E, and folate does not reduce the risk of lung cancer. *Am J Respir Crit Care Med., 177 (5),* 524-530.

Solomon, E.P., Berg, L.R., Matrin, D. W., & Villee, C. (1996). *Biology* (pp. 392-393, 802-812, 968, 1001, 1106). USA: Saunders College Publishing.

Statistical Solutions (n.d.). *Survival analysis with covariates*. Retrieved on March 15, 2011 at: http://www.statistical-solutions-software.com/BMDPdocuments/BMDP-2L.pdf

StatSoft (2010). *Electronic statistics textbook: Survival/failure time analysis.* Retrieved on March 15, 2011 at: http://www.statsoft.com/textbook/survival-failure-time-analysis/#rcoxwith

Sterner-Kock, A., Thorey, I. S., Koli, K., Wempe, F., Otte, J., Bangsow, T.,… von Melchner, H. (2002). Disruption of the gene encoding the latent transforming growth factor-beta binding protein 4 (LTBP-4) causes abnormal lung development, cardiomyopathy, and colorectal cancer. *Genes Dev., 16(17),* 2264 -2273

Sun, H., Nikolovska-Coleska, Z., Yang, C. Y., Qian, D., Lu, J., Qiu, S., Bai,… Wang, S. (2008). Design of small-molecule peptidic and nonpeptidic Smac mimetics. *Acc Chem Res., 41(10),* 1264-1277.

Takayama, H., Takakuwa, T., Dong, Z., Nonomura, N., Okuyama, A., Nagata, S., & Aozasa, K. (2001). Fas gene mutations in prostatic intraepithelial neoplasia and concurrent carcinoma: Analysis of laser capture microdissected specimens. *Lab Invest., 81(3),* 283-288.

The ATBC Cancer Prevention Study Group (1994). The Alpha-Tocopherol, Beta-Carotene Lung Cancer Prevention Study: Design, methods, participant characteristics, and compliance. *Ann Epidemiol*, 4, 1-10.

van Leeuwen, C. J., & Vermeire, T. G. (2007). *Risk assessment of chemicals: An introduction*. Netherlands: Springer.

Vitols, S., Peterson, C., Larsson, O., Holm, P., & Aberg, B. (1992). Elevated uptake of low density lipoproteins by human lung cancer tissue in vivo. *Cancer Res., 52(22),* 6244-6247.

Wajant, H. (2002). The Fas signaling pathway: More than a paradigm. *Science, 296 (5573),* 1635-1636.

Wassertheil-Smoller, S. (2004). *Biostatistics and epidemiology: A primer for health and biomedical professionals*. USA: Springer-Verlag New York, Inc.

Weaver. R. F., & Hedrick, Ph. W. (1997). *Genetics* (pp. 501-509). USA: Wm. C. Brown Publisher.

Wharton, K., & Derynck, R. (2009). TGFbeta family signaling: Novel insights in development and disease. *Development, 136 (22),* 3691-3697

Williams, J. C., Forster, L. A., Tull, S. P., Wong, M., Bevan, R. J., & Ferns, G. A. (1997). Dietary vitamin E supplementation inhibits thrombin-induced platelet aggregation, but not monocyte adhesiveness, in patients with hypercholesterolaemia. *Int J Exp Pathol., 78(4),* 259-266.

World Health Organization (WHO). (2008). *World cancer report 2008.* Switzerland: Boyle, P., & Levin, B. (Eds.)

World Health Organization (WHO). (2009). *Cancer (Fact sheet N°297).* Retrieved July 18, 2010 at: http://www.who.int/mediacentre/factsheets/fs297/en/index.html

Wrana, J. L. (2000). Crossing smads. *Sci. STKE, 2000 (23)*, p. re1. doi: 10.1126/stke.2000.23.re1

Wright, M. E., Mayne, S. T., Stolzenberg-Solomon, R. Z., Li, Z., Pietinen, P., Taylor, P. R.,… Albanes, D. (2004). Development of a comprehensive dietary antioxidant index and application to lung cancer risk in a cohort of male smokers. *Am J Epidemiol., 160(1),* 68-76.

Wright, S. C., Zheng, H., & Zhong, J. (1996). Tumor cell resistance to apoptosis due to a defect in the activation of sphingomyelinase and the 24 kDa apoptotic protease (AP24). *FASEB J., 10(2),* 325-332.

Yang, X., Khosravi-Far, R., Chang, H. Y., & Baltimore, D. (1997). Daxx, a novel Fas-binding protein that activates JNK and apoptosis. *Cell, 89 (7),* 1067-1076.

Ying, S. Y. (1987). Inhibins and activins: Chemical properties and biological activity. *Proc. Soc. Exp. Biol. Med., 186 (3),* 253-264.

Zhang, P., Liu, B., Jenkins, G. M., Hannun, Y. A., & Obeid, L. M. (1997). Expression of neutral sphingomyelinase identifies a distinct pool of sphingomyelin involved in apoptosis. *J Biol Chem., 272(15),* 9609-

9612.

Zhang, Q. (n.d.). *Center for dose response modeling: Overview*. Retrieved on March 11, 2011 at: http://www.thehamner.org/institutes-centers/center-for-dose-response-modeling/

ABOUT THE AUTHOR

Dr. Widad Akreyi is a health academic and a multi award-winning international humanitarian. She holds a master's degree in genetics and a PhD in global health and cancer epidemiology and serves as peer-reviewer for high-profile medical journals. An accomplished researcher, she has authored several books on global health and human rights approaches to history and culture. You can visit her at www.widad.org

Made in the USA
Middletown, DE
03 November 2026

36496629R00060